ATLAS OF

LAPAROSCOPIC AND

HYSTEROSCOPIC TECHNIQUES

FOR GYNECOLOGISTS

ATLAS OF

LAPAROSCOPIC AND

HYSTEROSCOPIC TECHNIQUES

FOR GYNECOLOGISTS

Second Edition

EDITED BY

TOGAS TULANDI MD, FRCSC, FACOG

Professor of Obstetrics and Gynecology
Director, Division Reproductive Endocrinology and Infertility
McGill University, Montreal, Quebec, Canada

WB SAUNDERS

London   Edinburgh   New York   Philadelphia   Sydney   Toronto

WB Saunders is an imprint of Harcourt Brace and Company Limited

Harcourt Brace and Company Limited   24–28 Oval Road
London NW1 7DX, UK

The Curtis Center
Independence Square West
Philadelphia, PA 19106–3399, USA

Harcourt Brace & Company
55 Horner Avenue
Toronto, Ontario M8Z 4X6, Canada

Harcourt Brace & Company, Australia
30–52 Smidmore Street
Marrickville, NSW 2204, Australia

Harcourt Brace & Company, Japan
Ichibancho Central Building, 22–1 Ichibancho
Chiyoda-ku, Tokyo 102, Japan

First published 1994
Second edition 1999

A catalogue record for this book is available from the British Library

ISBN 0-7020-2294-2

Typeset by J&L Composition Ltd, Filey, North Yorkshire
Printed and bound in Hong Kong.

To our family, teachers, colleagues, fellows, residents
and operating room staff

Togas Tulandi MD

CONTENTS

CONTRIBUTORS

MAURICE A. BRUHAT
Département de Gynécologie Obstetrique
et Reproduction Humaine,
Polyclinique de l'Hôtel Dieu,
Centre Hospitalier Universitaire,
Clermont-Ferrand,
France

MICHAEL CANIS
Département de Gynécologie Obstetrique
et Reproduction Humaine,
Polyclinique de l'Hôtel Dieu,
Centre Hospitalier Universitaire,
Clermont-Ferrand,
France

PAUL CARUANA
Department of Obstetrics and Gynaecology,
Universita Cattolica del Sacro Cuore,
Rome,
Italy

GIOVAN FIORE CATALANO
Department of Obstetrics and Gynaecology,
Universita Cattolica del Sacro Cuore,
Rome,
Italy

CHARLES CHAPRON
Clinique Universitaire Baudelocque,
Service de Chirurgie Gynécologique,
CHU Cochin Port Royal,
Paris,
France

JENNIFER Y. CLAMAN
Department of Obstetrics and Gynecology,
University College of Los Angeles,
California,
USA

STEPHEN L. CORSON
Women's Institute,
Philadelphia,
Pennsylvania,
USA

ALAN H. DeCHERNEY
Department of Obstetrics and Gynecology,
University College of Los Angeles,
California,
USA

JAN A. DEPREST
Department of Obstetrics and Gynaecology,
UZ Gasthuisberg,
Leuven,
Belgium

JEAN-BERNARD DUBUISSON
Clinique Universitaire Port Royal,
Service de Chirurgie Gynécologique,
CHU Cochin Port Royal,
Paris,
France

JOSEPH R. FESTE
Obstetrical and Gynecological Associates,
Houston,
Texas,
USA

HERVÉ FOULOT
Clinique Universitaire Baudelocque,
Service de Chirurgie Gynécologique,
CHU Chochin Port Royal,
Paris,
France

REINALDO GOLDCHMIT
Polyclinique Gynécologie Obstétrique,
Université de Clermont-Ferrand,
Médecine de la Reproduction,
Clermont-Ferrand,
France

ROGER HART
Minimally Invasive Therapy Unit and
Endoscopy Training Centre,
University Department of Obstetrics and
Gynaecology,
The Royal Free Hospital,
Hampstead,
London,
UK

NICHOLAS KADAR
Cranbury,
New Jersey,
USA

CHARLES H. KOH
Reproductive Speciality Center,
Milwaukee,
Wisconsin,
USA

THOMAS L. LYONS
Center for Women's Care and
Reproductive Surgery,
Atlanta,
Georgia,
USA

GÉRARD MAGE
Département de Gynécologie Obstetrique
et Reproduction Humaine,
Polyclinique de l'Hôtel Dieu,
Centre Hospitalier Universitaire,
Clermont-Ferrand,
France

ADAM MAGOS
Consultant Gynaecologist
Minimally Invasive Therapy Clinic,
Department of Obstetrics and Gynaecology,
The Royal Free Hampstead NHS Trust,
London,
UK

SALVATORE MANCUSO
Department of Obstetrics and
Gynaecology,
Universita Cattolica del Sacro Cuore,
Rome,
Italy

RICCARDO MARANA
Department of Obstetrics and Gynaecology,
Universita Cattolica del Sacro Cuore,
Rome,
Italy

PETER McCOMB
Department of Obstetrics and Gynecology,
University of British Columbia,
Vancouver Hospital,
Vancouver,
British Columbia
Canada

LISELOTTE METTLER
Department of Obstetrics and
Gynaecology,
University of Kiel,
Kiel,
Germany

LUDOVICO MUZII
Department of Obstetrics and
Gynaecology,
Universita Cattolica del Sacro Cuore,
Rome,
Italy

ROBERT S. NEUWIRTH
Director of Hysteroscopic Surgery
St Luke's Roosevelt Hospital Center,
New York,
New York,
USA

CAMRAN R. NEZHAT
Department of Surgery and
Department of Obstetrics and Gynecology
Endoscopy Center,
Stanford University School of Medicine,
Stanford,
California,
USA

CEANA H. NEZHAT
Department of Obstetrics and Gynecology,
Stanford University School of Medicine,
Palo Alto,
California,
USA

FARR R. NEZHAT
Department of Obstetrics and
Gynecology,
Stanford University School of Medicine,
Palo Alto,
California,
USA

JEAN LUC POULY
Département de Gynécologie Obstetrique
et Reproduction Humaine,
Polyclinique de l'Hôtel Dieu,
Centre Hospitalier Universitaire,
Clermont-Ferrand,
France

DAVID B. REDWINE
St Charles Medical Center,
Bend,
Oregon,
USA

CARLO ROMANINI
"Tor Vegata",
University of Rome,
Rome,
Italy

MAURIZIO ROSATI
Department of Obstetrics and Gynecology,
Stanford University School of Medicine,
Palo Alto,
California,
USA

DOMINIQUE VAN SCHOUBROECK
Department of Obstetrics and Gynaecology,
UZ Gasthuisberg,
Leuven,
Belgium

DANIEL S. SEIDMAN
Department of Obstetrics and Gynecology,
Stanford University School of Medicine,
Palo Alto,
California,
USA

KURT SEMM
5160 East Oakmont Drive,
Tuscon,
Arizona,
USA

EUGENIO SOLIMA
"Tor Vegata",
University of Rome,
Rome,
Italy

YUNG KUEI SOONG
Department of Obstetrics and Gynecology,
Chang Gung Memorial Hospital,
Kwei Shan,
Tao Yuan,
Taiwan

ERIC S. SURREY
Reproductive Medicine and Surgery
Associates,
Beverly Hills,
California,
USA

SALLI I TAZUKE
Department of Obstetrics and Gynecology,
Stanford University School of Medicine,
Palo Alto,
California,
USA

HOWARD C. TOPEL
1025 Summit,
Deerfield,
Illinois,
USA

TOGAS TULANDI
Department of Obstetrics and Gynecology,
McGill University,
Montreal,
Quebec,
Canada

RAFAEL F. VALLE
Department of Obstetrics and Gynecology,
Northwestern University Medical School,
Prentice Women's Hospital and Maternity
Center,
Chicago,
Illinois,
USA

KAMIEL VANDENBERGHE
Department of Obstetrics and Gynaecology,
UZ Gasthuisberg,
Leuven,
Belgium

YVES VILLE
Fetal Medicine Unit,
St George's Hospital Medical School,
London,
UK

ARNAUD WATTIEZ
Polyclinique Gynécologie Obstétrique,
Université de Clermont-Ferrand,
Médecine de la Reproduction,
Clermont-Ferrand,
France

WENDY K. WINER
Center for Women's Care and
Reproductive Surgery, and Emory
University School of Nursing,
Atlanta,
Georgia,
USA

ERRICO ZUPI
"Tor Vegata",
University of Rome,
Rome,
Italy

FOREWORD

Richard TeLinde in the early part of this century suggested that the reasons to operate were to save life, relieve suffering, and to correct significant anatomic abnormalities. Today we can add a fourth reason, to create life. The editor of this text has carefully adhered to these principles and devote significant discussion to preoperative evaluation and the appropriate selection of the patient for the correct operation.

A unique feature of this text is the concern expressed on "how to attain technological excellence" in the performance of a specific procedure. The training methods required as well as the specific instrumentation necessary to attain the desired result are carefully outlined.

This *Atlas of Laparoscopic and Hysteroscopic Techniques* is a superb addition to the medical literature. A truly international faculty of experienced surgeons have carefully described with detailed illustrations contemporary hysteroscopic, falloposcopic, and laparoscopic techniques. At a time when endoscopic techniques are rapidly expanding and have been introduced into gynecological practice worldwide, this *Atlas of Laparoscopic and Hysteroscopic Techniques* will serve as a welcome reference for gynecological surgeons.

John A. Rock MD

PREFACE

The continued advances in new technical skills require that such a book as the *Atlas of Laparoscopic Techniques* undergo updating. Indeed almost all procedures that previously required a laparotomy can now be done by endoscopy. As the field has expanded, several chapters such as laparoscopy in pregnancy, radical hysterectomy and endoscopic fetal surgery are added. Many colleagues and readers have also encouraged extension of this book to hysteroscopy. The format is concise, practical and step-by-step illustrations on how to perform a range of surgical interventions by endoscopy is maintained. The contributors are surgeons who have many years of experience in the procedures they describe.

In a similar way to the first edition, this book focuses on surgical technique. It is a book for student surgeons, residents, fellows and practising gynecologists. Some tips in this book will be helpful to facilitate the conduct of surgery either by laparoscopy or by hysteroscopy.

The author is grateful to the contributors, to Brenda Kennedy for her illustrations and to the staff of W.B. Saunders for their continuous support for both the first and this edition of the book and for their expertise in publishing medical works.

Togas Tulandi MD

BASIC PRINCIPLES OF LAPAROSCOPIC SURGERY

Togas Tulandi

Advances in technology including instrumentation and video-imaging have led to rapid progress in laparoscopic surgery. Accordingly, many procedures that previously required a laparotomy can be performed by laparoscopy. Operative laparoscopy, however, demands a higher degree of technical skills and a greater variety of equipment than for diagnostic laparoscopy or tubal sterilization. Knowledge of anatomy and pathology and the familiarity of the surgeon with the instruments are mandatory. Depending on the surgeon's preference, the procedure can be done with either laser, ultrasound scalpel, electrocautery or scissors.

SETUP

The setup should ideally involve two video monitor screens. The monitors are placed on each side of an assistant who stands at the end of the operating table between the patient's legs (Fig. 1.1). The surgeon stands facing one monitor on the opposite side and the assistant faces the second monitor. For one video monitor setup, the monitor is placed at the end of an operating table between the patient's legs for easy viewing by both the surgeon and the assistant (Figs 1.2 and 1.3). A surgical team that is familiar with operative laparoscopy is invaluable. They are responsible for the operation of monopolar or bipolar electrosurgical gener-

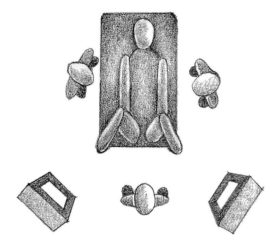

Figure 1.1 Operating room setup for two video monitors. The monitors are placed on each side of a second assistant who stands at the end of the operating table between the patient's legs. The surgeon stands facing one monitor on the opposite side and the first assistant faces the second monitor.

ators, laser and suction irrigator. They should be knowledgeable of all laparoscopic instruments and should know how to find a back-up instrument at short notice.

POSITIONING AND PREPARATION

Under low lithotomy position, the patient is placed horizontally until insertion of the laparoscope into the abdominal cavity. Using Allen stirrups or knee braces, the thighs are placed almost parallel to the abdomen (Fig. 1.4). This will facilitate manipulation of instruments. The lateral

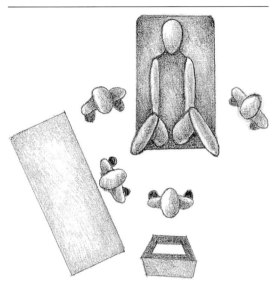

Figure 1.2 Operating room setup for one video monitor. The monitor is placed at the end of an operating table behind a second assistant. For easy viewing by both the surgeon and the first assistant, the second assistant should be sitting. The scrub nurse stands between the first and the second assistant and in front of the instrument table.

aspect of the knee should be well padded to prevent peroneal nerve compression. A rigid intrauterine cannula is inserted into the uterus to allow manipulation of the uterus and to permit chromopertubation. A disposable plastic intrauterine cannula is preferable. An intravenous line is inserted through the patient's arm on the assistant's side and the arm on the side of the operating surgeon should be placed by the patient's side and protected with an ulnar pad. An extended arm will interfere with the surgeon's mobility. Furthermore, brachial plexus neuropathy has been reported after laparoscopic surgery using a steep Trendelenburg position with shoulder braces and the patient's arm extended at 90°. To ascertain that the bladder is empty throughout the procedure, an indwelling catheter is placed inside the bladder and is removed at the end of the operation. When extensive adhesion or advanced endometriosis requiring extensive dissection in the vicinity of the large bowel is suspected, a bowel prep is indicated. A simple bowel prep is achieved by drinking 90 ml of a Phospha-soda solution the day before surgery. Shaving of the abdomen and pubic area is not required. Laparoscopy of the pelvic organs is done in the Trendelenburg position (about 30°).

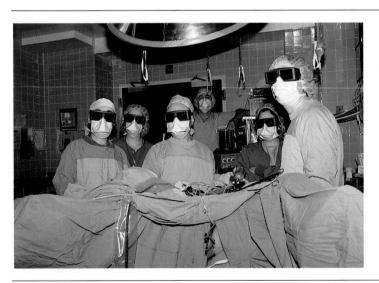

Figure 1.3 Laparoscopic surgery using a 3-D monitor. Special glasses are required to obtain three-dimensional perception of the image.

TROCAR INSERTION

The primary trocar is inserted via a 1 cm infraumbilical incision. Direct trocar insertion without the use of a Veress needle can be done using a disposable trocar. It has a retractable inner trocar and its tip is always sharp. In non-obese women, a Veress needle or primary trocar is inserted at 45° from horizontal. The aortic bifurcation in non-obese women is located about 0.4 cm cranial to the umbilicus. Because in obese women, the bifurcation is approximately 2.5 cm cranial to the umbilicus, the angle of insertion can be safely increased. In patients who have undergone multiple laparotomies, an open laparoscopy using a blunt trocar is recommended. A trocar sleeve loaded with a lapa- roscope is a simpler alternative to a blunt trocar. Pneumoperitoneum is achieved by insufflating the abdominal cavity with carbon dioxide (CO_2) gas. The gas is infused at a rate of 1–3 l/min and the intra-abdominal pressure should be below 20 mmHg. The abdomen is observed for global distension and the disappearance of liver dullness. Adequate pneumoperitoneum is usually obtained with 2–3 l of CO_2. After insertion of the laparoscope, the abdominal cavity should be first evaluated for possible inadvertent injury by Veress needle or trocar.

I routinely use two secondary 5 mm trocars. These trocars are inserted just above the pubic hairline, lateral to the deep epigastric vessels (Figs 1.5–1.7) or on the

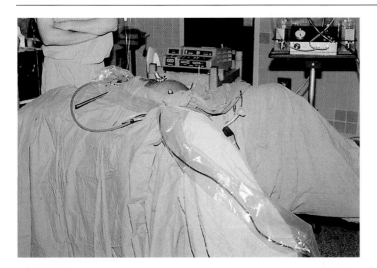

Figure 1.4 *The thighs are placed almost parallel to the abdomen. This will facilitate manipulation of the laparoscopic instruments.*

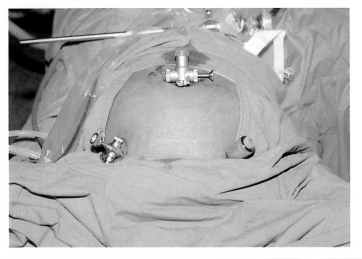

Figure 1.5 *Trocar sites.*

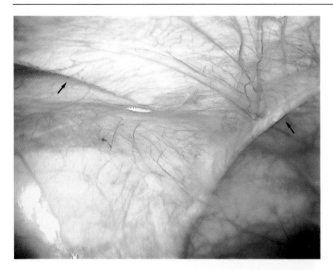

Figure 1.6 *Deep epigastric vessels* (left arrow) *are located lateral to the obliterated umbilical artery* (right arrow).

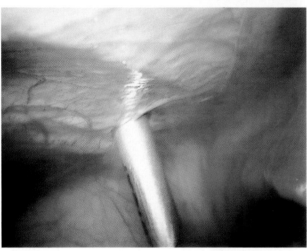

Figure 1.7 *Secondary trocar should be inserted under the laparoscopic control lateral to the deep epigastric vessels.*

midline. If removal of a specimen via the trocar is anticipated, one of the lateral trocars should be at least 10 mm. The trocars should always be inserted under direct laparoscopy control. The use of a forefinger as a guard to prevent too deep insertion is recommended (Fig. 1.8). Occasionally, another additional trocar is inserted on the midline between the two secondary trocars. During laparoscopy, the whole abdominal cavity including the upper abdomen should be inspected (Figs 1.9–1.12).

UNDER WATER INSPECTION

Near the completion of each laparoscopic procedure, irrigation of the abdominal cav-
ity should be performed and complete haemostasis is mandatory. Peritoneal lavage is done until the irrigating solution is free from blood and debris (Fig. 1.13). It should be noted that the pneumoperitoneum acts as a temporary tamponade and the bleeding may occur after the gas is evacuated from the abdominal cavity. Inspection of the operative field after instillation of approximately 500–1000 ml of Ringer's lactate ("examination under water") allows identification of bleeding points (Fig. 1.14). In a rat model, instillation of Ringer's lactate solution prevents adhesion formation.

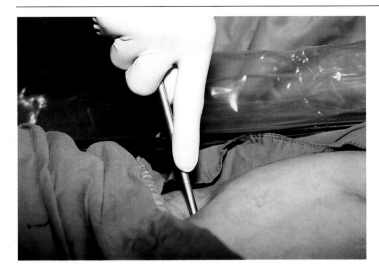

Figure 1.8 *A fore-finger is used to prevent deep insertion.*

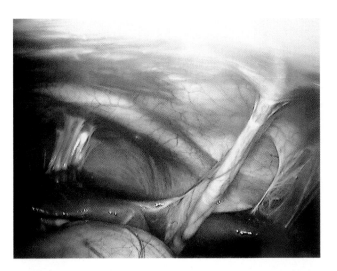

Figure 1.9 *The abdominal cavity including the upper abdomen should be systematically inspected. Here, perihepatic adhesions are seen.*

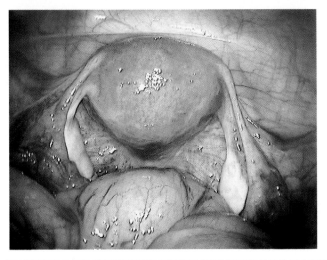

Figure 1.10 *Normal appearing pelvic organs.*

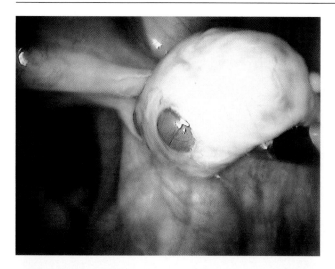

Figure 1.11 An exceptional finding of imminent ovulation.

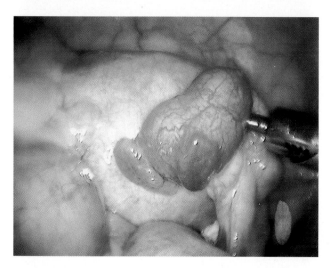

Figure 1.12 Accessory tubal ostium approximately 1 cm from the fimbriated opening.

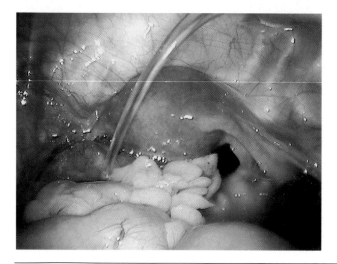

Figure 1.13 Instillation of crystalloid solution into the abdominal cavity.

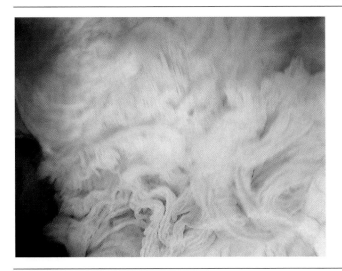

Figure 1.14 *"Examination under water" of normal fimbria.*

ANAESTHESIA

For operative laparoscopy, general anaesthesia with endotracheal intubation is mandatory. Assisting ventilation by mask before intubation may inflate the stomach and should be avoided. Otherwise, a nasogastric tube should be inserted to deflate the stomach before insertion of a Veress needle or a trocar. Shoulder braces may be needed for deep Trendelenburg position. Adequate ventilation is mandatory during the laparoscopic procedure. Rapid absorption of CO_2 gas and decrease of lung expansion due to the pneumoperitoneum and Trendelenburg position may result in hypercarbia. Cardiac arrythmias may then occur. If vasopressin is used, the anaesthetist should be notified before its administration. Although rare, its use has been associated with cardiac arrythmia and pulmonary oedema.

COMPLICATIONS AND THEIR PREVENTION

Injury to the deep epigastric vessels is avoided by transilluminating the abdominal wall before trocar insertion and by visualization of the vessels on the peritoneal surface of the anterior abdomen by the laparoscope. The vessels which are located lateral to the obliterated umbilical artery should be avoided (Fig. 1.6). Despite these measures, occasionally a large vessel is injured and brisk bleeding occurs. This can be controlled by a figure-of-eight suture with a retention suture or with a straight needle. Under direct laparoscopy control, a large needle through the whole thickness of the abdominal wall is placed with the trocar *in situ*. The trocar is then removed and the suture is tied. Another alternative is by using a Foley catheter. A no. 16 catheter is inserted into the abdominal cavity via the trocar. The balloon is inflated to 30 ml, the trocar is removed and the catheter is pulled outside until the balloon is tightly compressing the bleeding site. A clamp is placed on the outer side of the catheter at the skin level to maintain traction and haemostasis. The suture and the catheter are removed in 24 hours.

An incisional hernia may occur if the incision is ≥10 mm. A deep suture with 2-0 polyglycolic acid suture to approximate the fascia is required. This is needed particularly for a non-midline incision. Closure of this small incision is facilitated by the use of a sharply angled needle (U-shaped needle).

SUGGESTED READING

Hurd WH, Bude RO, DeLancey JOL, Pearl ML: The relationship of the umbilicus to the aortic bifurcation: implications for laparoscopic technique. *Obstet Gynecol* 1992 **80**: 48–51.

Tulandi T, Bugnah M: Operative laparoscopy: surgical modalities. *Fertil Steril* 1995 **63**: 237–245.

Tulandi T: Adhesion prevention in laparoscopic surgery. *Int J Fertil* 1996 **41**: 452–456.

Tulandi T, Beique F, Kimia M: Pulmonary edema: a complication of local injection of vasopressin at laparoscopy. *Fertil Steril* 1996 **66**: 478–480.

2

INSTRUMENTATION

Togas Tulandi and Liselotte Mettler

As any diagnostic laparoscopic intervention may turn into an operative procedure, basic laparoscopic instrumentation must always be available. Indeed, operative laparoscopy cannot be done adequately using standard equipment for diagnostic laparoscopy or for tubal sterilization. More equipment and a greater variety of instruments are needed. This chapter discusses basic operative laparoscopic instrumentation. Equipment that is already available for diagnostic laparoscopy or sterilization will not be discussed. It is crucial to have a good knowledge of the instruments. This will facilitate the conduct of surgery, and the instruments will be used wisely so that they will last longer. More importantly, the surgeon's familiarity with the instruments increases the safety of laparoscopic surgery. Beginners tend to purchase a wide variety of instruments that may or may not be eventually used. Furthermore, new instruments are being developed and tested continuously and some of them may replace the existing instruments. It is better to start with instruments described in this chapter and the set can be gradually expanded with instruments of your choice. The availability of good and well maintained laparoscopic instruments is invaluable. Back-up instruments are mandatory and should be available at short notice.

LAPAROSCOPE

A 10 mm straight forward 0° laparoscope has a large viewing angle. It is the best laparoscope for diagnostic as well as for operative surgery. A laparoscope with a laser channel is an alternative. The development of a smaller diameter laparoscope has renewed the interest in performing laparoscopy under local anaesthesia. The diameter of this minilaparoscope varies from 1.9 to 2.8 mm. Compared to a 10 mm laparoscope, visualization of the abdominal cavity is adequate but the image is smaller.

TROCARS AND REDUCER

Two trocars of 10 mm diameter and two or three trocars of 5 mm should be available. The secondary trocars are usually 5 mm, but one of them should be 10 mm or larger if removal of a specimen is anticipated. Here, a 10 to 5 mm reduction sleeve (reducer) is necessary (Fig. 2.1). For removal of large and solid specimen such as uterus or myoma, a 15 or 20 mm trocar to accommodate a morcellator is needed. An ultrashort reduction sleeve (3.75 cm) is also available.

The length of the trocar is usually 10.5 cm. Shorter trocars (5 cm) tend to slip from the abdominal cavity. It is desirable to have

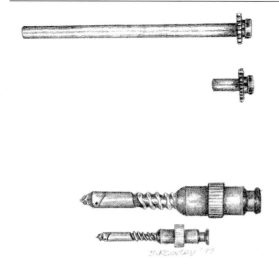

Figure 2.1 *Reduction sleeve. Short trocars with spiral threads.*

secondary trocars without valves. The valves interfere with insertion and removal of ancillary instruments, specimen or suture materials. Non-disposable trocars are more economical, but their sharpness should be maintained. Otherwise, disposable trocars should be used.

CAMERA AND MONITOR

These are mandatory for a safe conduct of operative laparoscopy. Maximum image quality can be obtained with the use of 3-chip-technology, high intensity light such as xenon or halogen light and a high resolution video monitor. A beamsplitter on the camera head for simultaneous viewing by endoscope and monitor screen decreases the amount of light and is not necessary. In fact, the use of a camera increases the safety of surgery. A video-recorder to record the conduct of surgery can be utilized for documentation and teaching. Photographs can be made using a video-printer.

Today, two-dimensional views and three-dimensional display technology capable of providing a clear and accurate sense of depth perception are available. The two-dimensional video images lack a true sense

of depth and may produce orientation difficulties for surgeons used to operating in opencases.However,experiencedendoscopic surgeons find that three-dimensional technology does not facilitate the conduct of surgery.

A mobile storage video-cart for the monitor, light source, insufflator, video-recorder or video-printer protects these expensive equipments from premature wear and tear and from accidents (Fig. 2.2).

HIGH FLOW INSUFFLATOR

Frequent instrument changes and constant irrigation and aspiration during a procedure lead to rapid loss of pneumoperitoneum. To maintain pneumoperitoneum, a high flow insufflator that administers up to 10 l of gas per minute is a prerequisite.

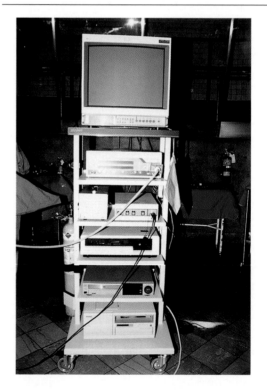

Figure 2.2 *A mobile storage video-cart for the monitor, insufflator, camera box, light source, video-recorder and video-printer.*

SUCTION-IRRIGATOR

A powerful irrigation pump that can deliver pressure of up to 800 mmHg is invaluable for operative laparoscopy. It is an efficient irrigator and it can also be used for hydro-dissection to separate tissue planes, adhesions, ovarian cyst wall or to flush products of conception out of the fallopian tube.

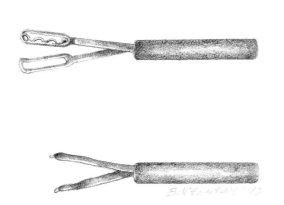

Figure 2.3 *Bipolar grasping forceps and microforceps.*

BIPOLAR AND UNIPOLAR INSTRUMENTS

A bipolar grasping forceps should always be available for haemostasis (Fig. 2.3). These are not replaceable by unipolar forceps or laser. A 5-mm bipolar microforceps allows accurate coagulation. Among unipolar instruments, unipolar scissors and a 1- mm needle electrode that can be inserted into a built-in channel suction-irrigator are invaluable (Fig. 2.4).

DISSECTING AND GRASPING FORCEPS

There are two types of grasping forceps: traumatic or atraumatic forceps (Fig. 2.5). For secure grasping, a 5-mm grasping forceps with 2 × 2 teeth can be used. A 10-mm claw forceps is useful for specimen removal (ovarian cyst, ovary, myoma etc.). Due to its powerful and sharp jaws, this forceps must only be applied to the tissue to be removed.

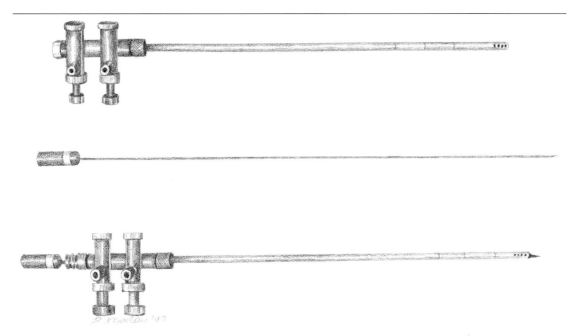

Figure 2.4 *Suction-irrigator: a unipolar needle electrode can be incorporated into the system.*

SCISSORS

Cold instruments including scissors remain the best tool for surgical dissection. A wide variety of scissors is available. The most commonly used scissors are shown in Fig. 2.6. It is important to have scissors that cut and do not tear the tissue. A combination of cutting and coagulating can be obtained by incorporating electrical energy to the scissors. An example is the unipolar Metzenbaum scissors. Because the scissors tend to become dull, frequent sharpening is necessary. Other types of scissors including hook scissors and microdissecting scissors should also be available.

SUTURE AND LIGATURE

Needle holders and suture forceps for a straight or ski needle and for a curved needle should be available (Fig. 2.7). The

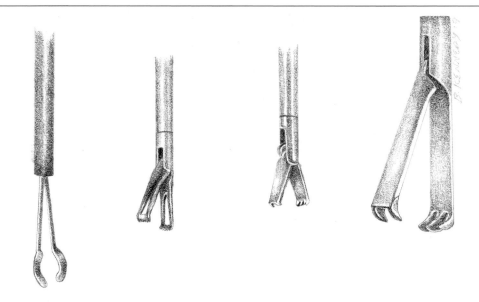

Figure 2.5 *Atraumatic grasping forceps, Babcock forceps, grasping forceps with teeth, 10-mm claw forceps.*

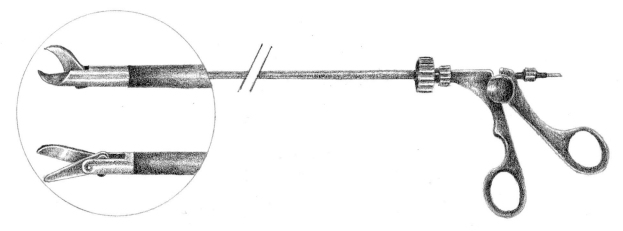

Figure 2.6 *Hook scissors and Metzenbaum scissors.*

use of a knot pusher (suture manipulator) allows extracorporeal tying and facilitates the procedure. The use of a non-disposable knot pusher with a fenestration at the end (Fig. 2.7) expedites the process of knot tying markedly. After suturing, the needle is extracted outside the abdominal cavity and inserted into the fenestration. The surgeon makes a knot and the knot is then pushed into the abdominal cavity. The procedure is repeated several times. Other types of knot pusher that do not have a fenestration require the surgeon to place the suture in the groove of the knotpusher. This takes time especially in a darkened operating theatre. The availability of a pretied ligature (Endoloops, Rx Ethicon Inc., Sommerville, NJ; PercLoop, Laparomed, Irvine, CA) per-mits easy ligature of structures including appendix, fallopian tube, ovary or a pedun-culated myoma.

MORCELLATOR

Occasionally, a morcellator is needed to reduce a large specimen such as myoma to small pieces allowing easy removal. The best morcellator is a serrated edge macro-morcellator (Fig. 2.8). It is available in manual and electric or battery-operated versions.

MISCELLANEOUS

Administration of a dilute solution of vaso-pressin decreases bleeding from the site of

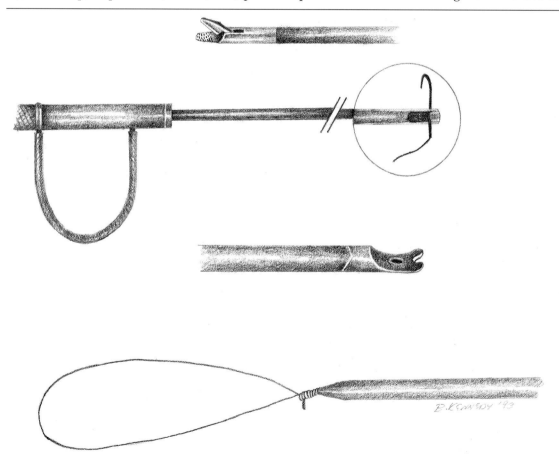

Figure 2.7 Needle holder for straight or ski needle, needle holder for curved needle, suture manipula-tor (knot pusher) with a fenestration and pretied ligature (loop).

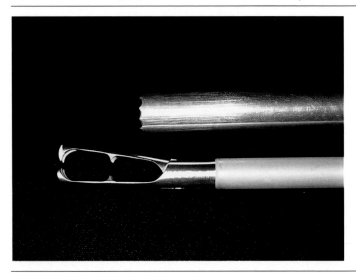

Figure 2.8 *Serrated edge macromorcellator and a claw forceps.*

tubal anastomosis, ectopic pregnancy or myomectomy. A spinal needle can be used, but it is not rigid and bends easily. A non-disposable injection needle (shaft diameter, 5 mm) that can be inserted via a secondary trocar is a better instrument. Stabilizing a myoma during dissection and enucleation can be achieved using a 5 or 10 mm cork screw. Although, they are not essential, a clip and a staple applicator might be needed.

LASER

Laser, electrocautery, ultrasound scalpel or regular scissors are merely surgical modalities. The clinical results depend more on the surgeon's experience and preference and proper patient selection.

DISPOSABLE INSTRUMENTS

There are many disposable instruments available. The use of non-disposable instruments is economical, but disposable instruments should be available in the operating theatre as back-up.

BASIC INSTRUMENTS

This is a list of the basic instruments. Back-up instruments are desirable.

1. A 10-mm straightforward laparoscope 0°.
2. Trocars:
   (a) 10-mm primary trocar,
   (b) 10-mm secondary trocar,
   (c) 5-mm secondary trocars (at least three),
   (d) 20-mm trocar for a morcellator.
3. 10 to 5 mm and 20 to 10 mm reduction sleeves.
4. Suction irrigation system.
5. Bipolar forceps with cable:
   (a) bipolar grasping forceps,
   (b) bipolar microforceps.
6. Unipolar instruments with cable:
   (a) 1-mm needle electrode,
   (b) unipolar scissors.
7. Forceps:
   (a) atraumatic grasping forceps,
   (b) 5-mm grasping forceps with 2 × 2 teeth (at least two),
   (c) 10-mm claw forceps.
8. Scissors:
   (a) Metzenbaum rotating forceps,
   (b) hook scissors,
   (c) microdissecting scissors.
9. Suture and ligature:
   (a) needle holder for straight or ski needle,
   (b) needle holder for curved needle,
   (c) assistant needle holder,
   (d) suture manipulator (knot pusher).

10. Miscellaneous:
    (a) 5-mm injection needle,
    (b) morcellator,
    (c) pretied ligature.

SUGGESTED READING

Hasson HM: Open laparoscopy: a report of 150 cases. *J Reprod Med* 1974 **12**: 234–238.

Reich H: New laparoscopic techniques. In Sutton C and Diamond MP (eds) *Endoscopic Surgery for Gynaecologists*. W.B. Saunders, London, 1993, pp. 28–39.

Tulandi T, Bugnah M: Operative laparoscopy: surgical modalities. *Fertil Steril* 1995 **63**: 237–245.

3

LAPAROSCOPIC SUTURING: EXTRACORPOREAL KNOT TYING

Peter McComb

The ability to place sutures by laparoscopy has facilitated procedures such as oophorectomy, salpingectomy, adnexectomy and many others. For these procedures the suture sizes have been 4-0 or heavier. These large suture sizes have limitations for reconstructive pelvic surgery because such suture material, as a residual foreign body, will induce adhesion formation. Otherwise, surgery by laparoscopy fulfils the prerequisites of the microsurgical approach with constant temperature, humidity, reduced peritoneal injury, magnification, and, when performed carefully, gentle tissue handling. Thus, the ability to use microsuture of size 6-0 or less, completes the prerequisites for a true "microsurgical approach" by laparoscopy.

The distinct advantage of the technique is the extracorporeal tying of the knot. Attempts to knot-tie microsuture within the peritoneal cavity are hampered by the abdominal wall, since it acts as a fulcrum for each of the instruments. The surgeon is thereby forced to use the short end of the lever to create motion at the long end of the lever; this is a disadvantage when the aim is to achieve small precise movements at the long end of the lever. Furthermore, intracorporeal knot formation with microsuture is made difficult by the attraction of the suture to peritoneal surfaces by fluid surface

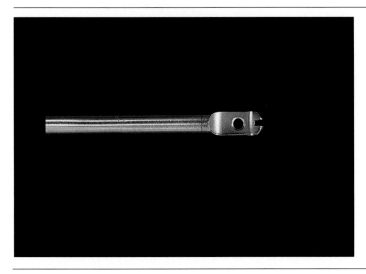

Figure 3.1 *A knot pusher or a suture manipulator.*

tension. It has to be performed gently, otherwise extracorporeal knot tying with fine sutures can be complicated by breakage of the sutures. Accordingly, some surgeons prefer the intracorporeal technique.

In order to perform an extracorporeal knot tying, a particular form of knot pusher is necessary (Fig. 3.1).

TECHNIQUE

1. The needle and suture are introduced into the peritoneal cavity with a 3-mm diameter needle driver grasping the suture approximately 1 cm from the needle (Fig. 3.2). Once in the pelvic cavity, the suture and needle are detached from the needle driver by placing the needle on the uterine serosa. The surface tension of the peritoneal fluid retains the needle. It is then picked up in the jaws of the driver (Fig. 3.3).

2. The needle is passed through the tissues. The needle is then drawn from the peritoneal cavity with the needle driver.

3. The throws of the knot are completed extracorporeally. After each throw, one end of the suture is threaded into the open end of the suture manipulator and out of the fenestration (Fig. 3.4). The other end of the suture remains free.

4. Equal tension is next applied to both ends of the suture, and the knot is slid down the length of the suture to apply it

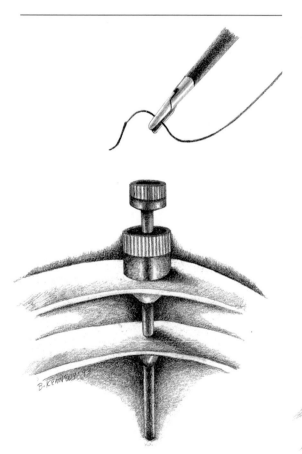

Figure 3.2 The needle is introduced into the peritoneal cavity by grasping the suture approximately 1 cm from the needle.

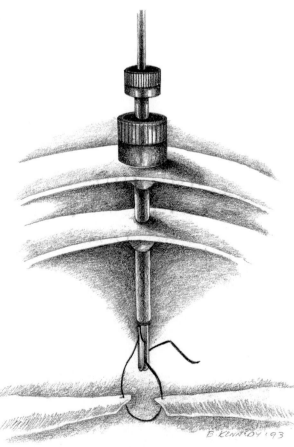

Figure 3.3 Withdrawing the suture from the peritoneal cavity by grasping it as in Fig. 3.2.

to the tissue (Fig. 3.5). This process is repeated to complete a surgical knot. Scissors placed through the additional port then cut the suture, and the loose suture ends are withdrawn. With experience, each suture takes only a few minutes to place.

APPLICATIONS OF EXTRACORPOREAL MICROSUTURE

The use of this technique brings remarkable versatility to the laparoscopic surgeon.

Examples are as follows.

- An ovary can be translocated and sutured extrapelvically to avoid radiation.
- The ovarian ligament can be sutured to the round ligament to preclude adhesion reformation.
- After ovarian cystectomy the ovarian cortex can be closed microsurgically.
- The fallopian tube can be anastomosed.
- Terminal salpingostomy can be stabilized better than without suture.
- Bowel and bladder injuries can be closed with lightweight sutures.
- Points of haemorrhage from precarious sites, such as bowel, or adjacent to the ureter may be secured more safely than with electrocoagulation.

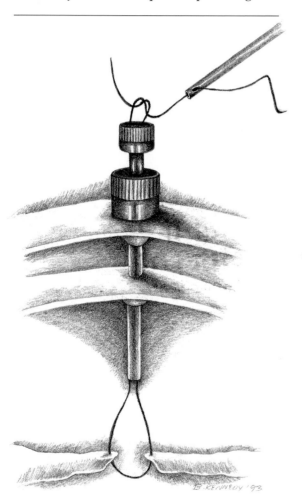

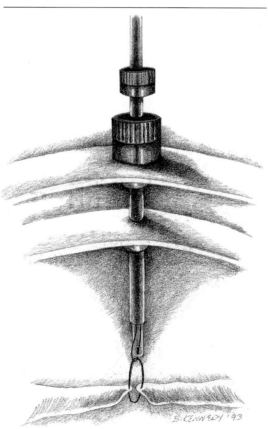

Figure 3.4 *The needle is inserted into the fenestration of the knot pusher before sliding the knot down into the peritoneal cavity.*

Figure 3.5 *Equal tension is applied to both ends of the suture and the knot is tightened with the help of the knot pusher.*

- Haemorrhage from an ovary that is diffuse can be stopped with an encircling stitch.
- A twisted adnexum, ovary or fallopian tube, once untwisted can be sutured to the pelvic sidewall to prevent futher torsion.
- The mesosalpinx of a well-vascularized ectopic pregnancy can be undersewn prophylactically before salpingotomy to remove the pregnancy tissues. (An isthmic ectopic pregnancy with a human chorionic gonadotropin level of 108, 631 IU/ml was successfully managed in this fashion).

POTENTIAL COMPLICATIONS AND THEIR PREVENTION

1. The needle may traumatize a vessel or bowel. However, its diameter is similar to a 30-gauge needle and is unlikely to require anything more than pressure on the vessel, or close examination of the bowel. The needle should pierce the bowel cleanly rather than cause a laceration. To avoid these inadvertent injuries, the operator must watch the needle at all times when it is mounted in the driver.

2. The suture and or needle may be lost. It is rare to lose a needle intraperitoneally. The magnification and illumination afforded by the laparoscope minimize this occurrence. Usually, the needle is found within the trocar sleeve; typically, it is either located within the trap or impaled on a rubber washer. Should the needle be lost absolutely then radiological localization and use of an intraperitoneal magnetized probe is required.

3. A loop of bowel can be entrapped by a space created by the sutured tissue. Such a space should be closed.

CONTRAINDICATIONS

There are many fertility promoting operations that may use microsuture. However, in our hands most anastomotic operations that join tubes are best performed by laparotomy rather than laparoscopy.

SUGGESTED READING

McComb PF: A new suturing instrument that allows the use of microsuture at laparoscopy. *Fertil Steril* 1992 **57**: 936–938.

4

LAPAROSCOPIC SUTURING: INTRACORPOREAL KNOT TYING

Howard C. Topel

Laparoscopic suturing is an endoscopic skill necessary for the successful performance of a variety of advanced and complex laparoscopic operations. Although some attempt to dismiss endosuturing as unnecessary, most experienced endoscopic surgeons recognize that neither energy sources, clips, nor stapling devices can replace the need for suturing. As with conventional open surgery, laparoscopic suturing techniques permit restoration of normal anatomical relationships, organ reconstruction, approximation of tissue planes, and the establishment of haemostasis. Of the three suturing and knot-tying methods (endoloop, extracorporeal and intracorporeal) adapted for laparoscopic surgery, the intracorporeal method remains the most difficult to master. Intracorporeal suturing is defined as the placement of suture and subsequent tying of a secure suture knot within the peritoneal cavity.

Once limited to only short straight or ski needles, endosuturing can now be performed with a variety of curved needles and different suture materials. The ability to utilize curved needle suturing provides the surgeon with greater operative flexibility, and permits easier adaptation to a two-dimensional video working field. Straight needles may appear to be more user friendly, but approximation of a deep myoma bed, or control of bleeding along the pelvic side wall requires the inherent advantages of a curved suture needle. Early

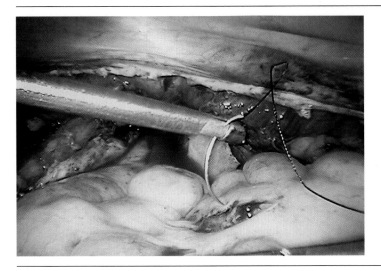

Figure 4.1 *Suturing using a curved needle.*

needle holders were designed only to grasp straight needles, which made their adaptation to curved suturing very inadequate. However, new curved needle drivers have been designed to firmly hold the needle with minimal instability at the tip (Fig. 4.1). This permits curved needles (i.e. SH, CT-3) to be driven through tissue of varying thickness and consistency. In addition, the suture needle can be precisely positioned and passed through tissue with a rotational motion similar to open laparotomy suturing.

INSERTION OF NEEDLE AND SUTURE INTO THE ABDOMINAL CAVITY

1. Advance the curved needle driver through the 10-mm suture introducer channel (Fig. 4.2).

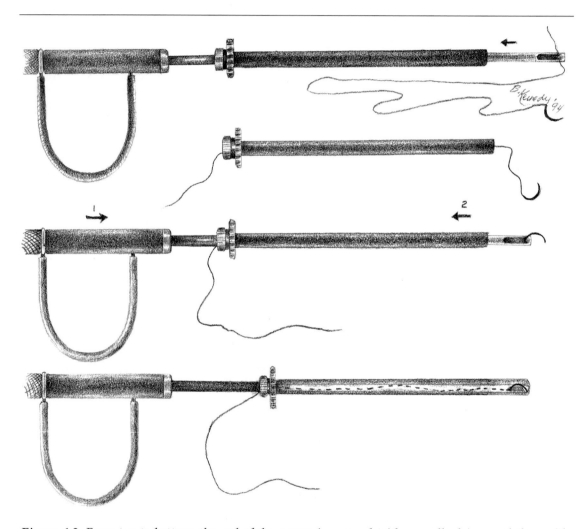

Figure 4.2 *From top to bottom: the end of the suture is grasped with a needle driver and then withdrawn into the introducer until it is completely outside the introducer. The needle holder is reinserted into the introducer (1) and the needle is positioned to allow withdrawal of the loaded needle driver into the introducer (2). This loaded introducer can now be inserted into the abdominal cavity and is ready to be used.*

2. Grasp the tail end of the suture in the needle driver jaws.

3. Pull the needle driver back through the suture introducer, allowing the suture needle (SH, CT-3) to hang freely beyond the end of the introducer (Fig. 4.2).

4. Release the suture from the jaws of the needle driver.

5. While stabilizing the suture line inside the channel, advance the needle driver back down the introducer.

6. Secure the suture needle (at the needle–suture junction) in the needle driver jaws, keeping the needle curve parallel to the driver and suture introducer.

7. Pull the suture taut (not tight). Then, withdraw the loaded needle driver into the introducer until the entire suture needle is inside the distal end.

8. Cut the excess suture, leaving approximately 25 mm or less exposed at the proximal end of the introducer. The critical suture length is 80–90 mm.

9. Re-advance the loaded introducer through the 10/11-mm trocar into the abdominal cavity (Fig. 4.2).

10. Following needle placement into the tissue, bring the entire length of suture into the abdominal cavity, and equalize the length of the suture ends in preparation for tying.

11. For needle removal, grasp the suture within the jaws of the needle driver 20 mm from the needle. Then cut the suture, and withdraw the needle into the introducer channel (Fig. 4.3).

12. The needle driver, suture needle and introducer are withdrawn all at once through the trocar port, leaving the trocar in place.

13. The suture is now ready for intra-abdominal knot-tying.

A second method of needle/suture introduction is to load the suture into the jaws of a needle driver approximately 2–3 cm behind the swage point. The needle driver and suture are introduced into a 10–12 mm trocar and advanced down into the abdominal cavity (Fig. 4.4).

An alternative to this technique is to remove the trocar from the abdominal wall and cover the open port site with a finger in order to avoid loss of the pneumoperitoneum. By grasping the suture near the swage, the needle driver can be backloaded into the trocar sheath. The trocar is then reintroduced, carrying the needle driver and suture, into the abdominal cavity. After the stitch has been placed, the needle can be removed by cutting the suture 2–3 cm from the swage. Re-grasp the short suture tail and pull the free needle into the trocar sheath. Withdraw the entire trocar out of the abdominal wall, as a finger is placed over the trocar site to prevent loss of

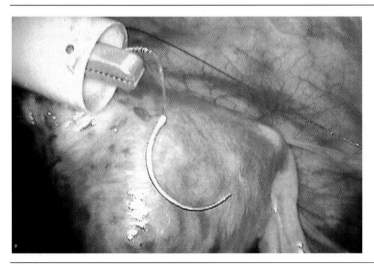

Figure 4.3 *Removal of the needle by grasping the suture with a needle driver approximately 20 mm from the needle and then withdrawing into the introducer.*

pneumoperitoneum. After the needle is removed from the trocar sheath, the trocar can be reinserted into the abdominal cavity under direct vision.

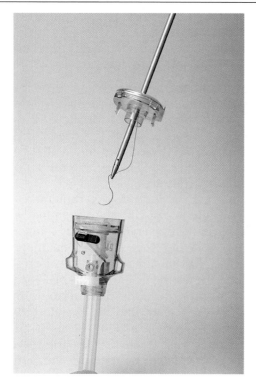

Figure 4.4 The needle driver and suture are first introduced into a trocar and then advanced into the abdominal cavity.

These various needle/suture introduction and retrieval techniques are designed to visualize and control the curved needle at all times, in order to prevent inadvertent tissue injury or loss of the needle within the abdominal cavity.

KNOT TYING

Intracorporeal knot-tying can be a tedious, time consuming, and often demanding experience. However, with patience and a great amount of practice, intra-abdominal knot-tying can be mastered, and become a valuable endoscopic skill. There are two types of intracorporeal knot-tying: classic instrument tie and a "twist" technique.

Classic technique

The classic instrument knot-tying technique is similar to that performed during open laparotomy surgery. The needle is not removed before knot tying and is used to control the suture line. Formation of loops is facilitated by holding the tip of the needle with one of the needle drivers (Fig. 4.5).

"Twist" technique

A "twist" knot-tying technique simplifies endoscopic suture tying. This technique is

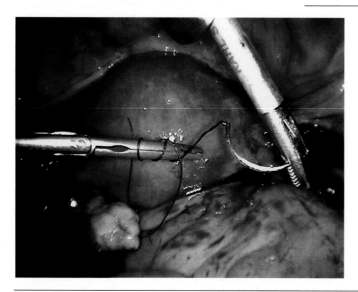

Figure 4.5 Knot tying is facilitated by holding the tip of the needle with one of the needle drivers.

illustrated in Fig. 4.6. It is applicable to all suture sizes and is designed to consistently form a square double "surgeon" knot with minimal slippage. One end of the suture is rotated up the shaft of a 5-mm grasping instrument until three or four loops are formed. A second grasper removes the suture end from the jaws of the rotating grasper, and slides the end upward along the shaft. The other free suture end is now grasped by the first grasper. As both instruments are pulled in opposite directions, a square double knot is formed. The knot can be tightened against the tissue surface and will not loosen as a second knot is similarly fashioned and positioned onto the tissue.

This "twist" technique provides excellent approximation of heavy tissue under tension, such as with uterine reconstruction following myomectomy. In addition, fine microsurgical knot-tying with delicate suture is readily accomplished with this technique. The "twist" knot-tie is a reliable and consistent way to form a non-slipping knot and establish haemostasis.

CONTINUOUS SUTURE

Laparoscopic surgery does not preclude the ability to perform continuous endosuturing.

1. With the aid of a specially designed applier (Fig. 4.7), a PDS clip, called a

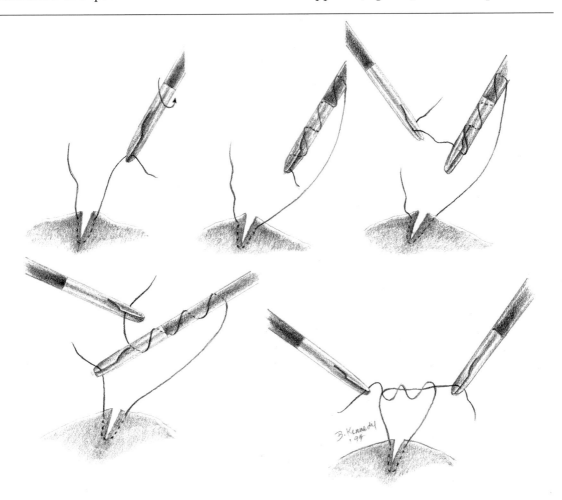

Figure 4.6 Knot-tying with a "twist" technique.

"Laparo-tye", can be attached to the suture end. One clip serves to anchor the start of the suture line, while a second PDS clip secures the continuous locking closure. This continuous technique, employing PDS clips, approximates a large uterine defect following myomectomy with an excellent anatomical reconstruction.

2. A second continuous suture technique can be performed with the formation of a slip knot at the free end. After the needle is initially passed through the tissue, the needle and suture line is passed through the loop and pulled tight, locking the knot against the tissue (Fig. 4.8). After the continuous closure is completed, the final knot is made with a classic or "twist" knot-tying technique.

With the continuous advancement toward performing more difficult operations, the necessity for improved laparoscopic suturing skills is crucial. Endosuturing will not only permit the correct execution of the operation, but will help to minimize the potential for postoperative complications. Furthermore, when complications do occur, endosuturing techniques will be available to repair a bowel laceration, to close an inad-

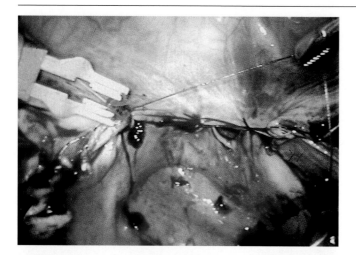

Figure 4.7 *Continuous suturing with the help of a "Laparo-tye" to anchor the beginning of the suture line.*

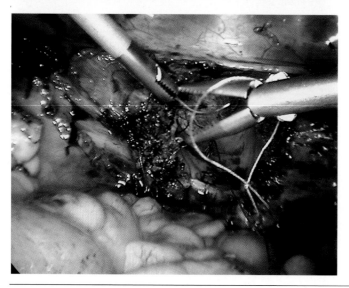

Figure 4.8 *Continuous suturing technique using a slip knot on its free end.*

vertent cystotomy, or to selectively ligate a bleeding vessel near the ureter. Only great patience and hours of dedicated practice will allow the laparoscopic surgeon to develop the dexterity, and to gain the confidence to perform endosuturing. However, once mastered, laparoscopic suturing will permit the successful completion of complex operations with fewer complications, and with surgical results that meet the expectations of open laparotomy surgery.

5

LYSIS OF ADHESIONS

Peter McComb

SALPINGO-OVARIOLYSIS

Preliminary assessment of the pelvis is key to successful salpingo-ovariolysis. Vital structures including bowel, vessels, bladder and ureter and their involvement in the distorted anatomy are identified at the outset. Adhesions obscure structures and proximity of the peritoneum (and vessels and ureter) to the scar tissue makes differentiation between the two difficult.

After establishing the pneumoperitoneum, omentum may be seen to be adhered to the anterior abdominal wall and to the pelvis. It is often necessary to remove the omental adhesions from the abdominal wall before the pelvic contents can be fully visualized. Trocars are inserted at a distance and angle optimal for lysis of the omentum. Electrocautery and scissors are best suited to this type of lysis. The omentum tends to revascularize surrounding adherent organs. Unless cautery is used, omental vessels characteristically retract and continue to bleed. If adhesions exist between omentum and the pelvis, the same scissor/electrocautery lysis is best.

After preliminary removal of any omental adhesions, the uterus is mobilized with an intracervical cannula. The patient is placed in the Trendelenburg position and bowel is displaced towards the upper abdomen. This may be hampered by adhesions between bowel and the pelvis. Trocars are placed about two finger breadths above the pubic symphysis. One midline and two lateral trocars are usually needed. Probes and atraumatic grasping forceps are inserted to angulate the various organs so as to assess the full extent and type of adhesions, and to identify the organs involved.

In principle, it is better to excise scar tissue. If the adherent structure (such as omentum) will be displaced some distance after incision of the adhesion, then excision of adhesions is unnecessary. If there is fusion of two organs, excision of the scar is not possible.

There are three commonly used forms of incision: scissors, electrocautery and CO_2 laser. Unipolar electrocautery has a thermal shoulder of lateral spread of heat of greater than 2 mm; CO_2 laser has a shoulder of at least 1 mm and scissors have none. This allows close dissection to vital structures and to the delicate tissues of the tubes and ovaries. Another instrument, the "aquapurator" can deliver lactated Ringers solution at pressures of 100 mmHg to the adherent tissues.

There are two basic forms of adhesions: those that are dense and fibrous, often involving a large surface area of the respective organs, and those that are filmy, flimsy and may be transparent. Lysis of these two types of adhesion from the pelvic organs presents unique problems.

OVARIOLYSIS

The ovary has a single-cell layer surface epithelium. Loss of this epithelium predisposes to scar formation. The ovary itself should not be grasped if at all possible.

Filmy adhesions

These are typically between tube, bowel, omentum and peritoneum and ovary. Traction is placed on the scar tissue with grasping forceps at the scar attachment away from the ovary. The adhesion is angled opti-mally for incision (Fig. 5.1). Scissors are used to incise the adhesion at the level of the ovarian surface (Fig. 5.2). There is no serosa to tent up from the ovary, and complete removal of the scar will facilitate ovulation. Some practitioners advocate laser or electrocautery. Any bleeding will almost always subside spontaneously. If not, vasopressin solution (0.5 units/ml normal saline) injected interstitially will assist. Electrocoagulation with fine pronged bipolar forceps may be needed. This is usually held in reserve. Alternatively, 6-0 suture can be used to achieve haemostasis.

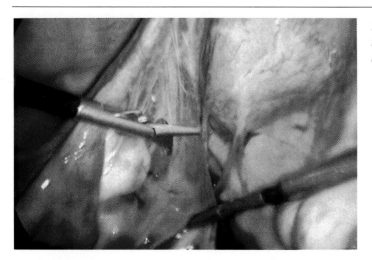

Figure 5.1 *The adhesion is stretched with a grasping forceps and then divided with scissors.*

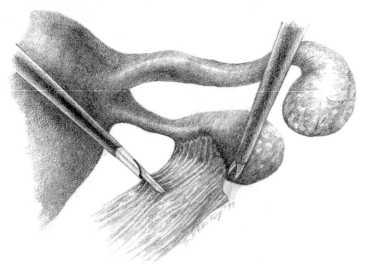

Figure 5.2 *Cutting of adhesions at the level of the ovarian surface.*

Dense adhesions

Adhesions of the ovary to the pelvis, bowel to ovary, hydrosalpinx or ampulla to ovary often result in dense, fibrous scarring. In these instances, mechanical lysis of the adhesions is the most effective modality. Sharp incision is followed by use of the aquapurator (hydrodissector) to establish the cleavage plane (Fig. 5.3). The aquapurator rinses the tissues from serosanguinous fluid and assists in visualization.

If the extensive raw surfaces created by the adhesiolysis are allowed to simply fall together at the conclusion of the adhesiolysis, then scar reformation is inevitable. Use of 6-0 polypropylene suture to suture one organ away from another is useful. Floatation of the pelvic organs by leaving 1000 ml of lactated Ringer's solution in the pelvis also mitigates reformation of the scarring. For example, if an ovary affected by endometriosis has been dissected from the ovarian fossa with the creation of raw tissue surfaces, then the ovary may be elevated by suturing the ovarian ligament to the round ligament. To accomplish this, 6-0 suture is passed through the round ligament,

through the mesosalpinx (elevate the tubal isthmus and identify an avascular window), through the ovarian ligament and back again to the round ligament to be tied (Figs 5.4 and 5.5).

SALPINGOLYSIS

Filmy adhesions

Any of the pelvic contents may be attached by filmy, flimsy transparent scarring to the oviduct. These have the potential to prevent oocyte retrieval by creating a barrier between tube and ovary and by limiting the motion of the fimbria and the exposure of the tube to the ovulated oocyte. Fortunately, such adhesions are readily lysed with a low attendant risk of reformation.

Any of the three incisional modalities may be used to incise the adhesions. A peculiarity of the fallopian tube is the loose serosa that invests the myosalpinx. When traction is applied to the scar, the serosa is tented upwards (Fig. 5.6). Care is needed to avoid incision of the serosa with denudation of the oviduct. Make sure that the incisions are placed at a distance from the serosa.

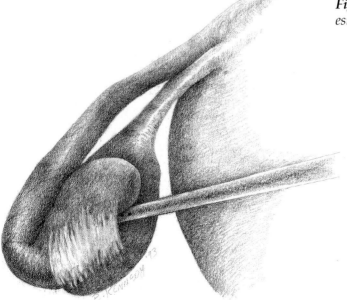

Figure 5.3 *Hydrodissection is used to establish a cleavage plane.*

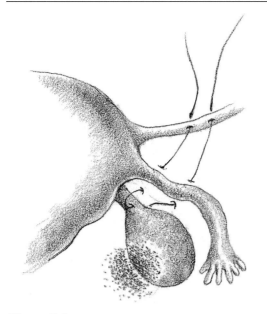

Figure 5.4

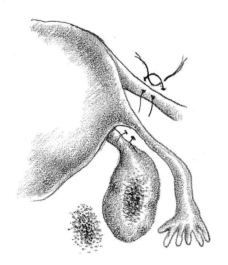

Figure 5.5

Figure 5.4 and Figure 5.5 *Suturing the ovarian ligament to the round ligament by passing 6-0 suture through the round ligament, through the mesosalpinx (elevate the tubal isthmus and identify an avascular window), through the ovarian ligament and back again to the round ligament.*

Dense adhesions

The tubal ampulla and hydrosalpinx are often densely adherent to the ovary. The scarring is not only dense but vascular. When the hydrosalpinx is adherent, it is necessary to distend the tube with dye solution to determine which part of the hydrosalpinx is fused to the ovary. It is usually the terminal portion of the tube. This tubal tissue should be preserved carefully if tubal function is to occur.

Ampullary–ovarian scarring is best approached by commencing the dissection from the midsection of the tube towards the fimbria (Fig. 5.7). In both instances mechanical lysis is the best. Where it is clear that there is substantial vascularity, it is prudent to have the vasopressin solution at hand.

Injection of the dye solution may leak from the hydrosalpinx into the mesosalpinx so that the mesosalpinx mimics the terminal portion of the tube. If this is not recognized, the mesosalpinx will be incised with subsequent haemorrhage. In this situation bipolar cautery and/or 6-0 polypropylene will be necessary.

POTENTIAL COMPLICATIONS AND THEIR PREVENTION

Haemorrhage is the most likely complication associated with salpingo-ovariolysis. The ability to use bipolar and unipolar electrocautery and suture at laparoscopy are key to the control of haemorrhage. The prevention of bleeding stems from an education in laparoscopic anatomy. Judicious prophylactic use of cautery, suture and vasopressor solution also assist in certain cases.

RESULTS

Lysis of adhesions to treat infertility is variably successful. The outcome depends on the extent of the scarring and the likelihood of scar reformation. Scarring as a consequence of previous surgery or endometriosis is especially difficult to treat without reoccurrence. Optimal prospects for pregnancy, with rates in excess of 50%, are yielded typically in cases where the adhesions are filmy and extensive but readily amenable to lysis.

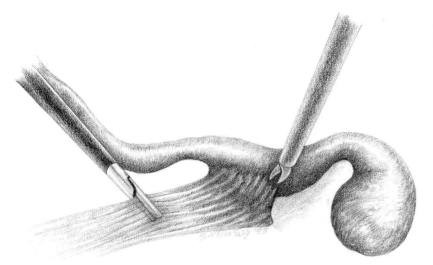

Figure 5.6 *Cutting peritubal adhesions. Note that the serosa of the tube is tented.*

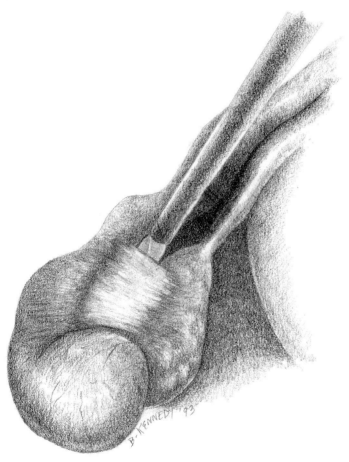

Figure 5.7 *Dissection of ampullary–ovarian adhesions from the midsection of the tube towards the fimbria.*

CONTRAINDICATIONS

1. If the salpingo-ovariolysis will not improve the fertility then it should not be performed. Such cases include dense adhesions and scarring that involves extensive fusion of the peritoneal organs.
2. Proximity of the bowel, bladder and ureter to the adhesions are relative contraindications especially in dense extensive scarring.
3. Genital tract tuberculosis is an absolute contraindication.

SUGGESTED READING

Gomel V. (ed): *Microsurgery in Female Infertility*, Little, Brown, Boston, PA, 1983.

McComb P: Infertility surgery: operative endoscopy, new instruments and techniques. *Clin Obstet Gynecol* 1989 **32**: 564–575.

6

DISTAL TUBAL DISEASE: SALPINGOSTOMY AND FIMBRIAL PHIMOSIS REPAIR

Peter McComb

SALPINGOSTOMY

The advent of laparoscopically directed salpingostomy allows the surgery to be performed at the time of the assessment of the hydrosalpinx at laparoscopy. As the oviduct is assessed, associated proximal tubal disease is identified. Frequently, there are peritubal and periovarian adhesions tethering the hydrosalpinx to the ovary, and the ovary to the pelvic sidewall and other pelvic structures such as bowel and uterus. These adhesions can be excised by scissors, electro-cautery or CO_2 laser before repairing the hydrosalpinx.

Procedure

1. Grasping forceps with a "diamond shaped jaw" are placed on the distal ampulla of the tube, immediately adjacent to the hydrosalpinx. The hydrosalpinx is distended with transcervical dye solution and the pattern of scarring is observed (Fig. 6.1).

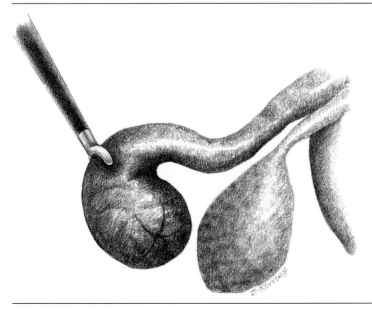

Figure 6.1 Chromopertubation with solution of methylene blue distending the hydrosalpinx. Note the pattern of scarring.

Figure 6.2a

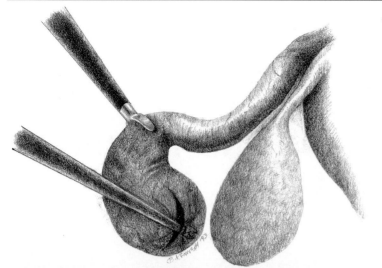

Figure 6.2b

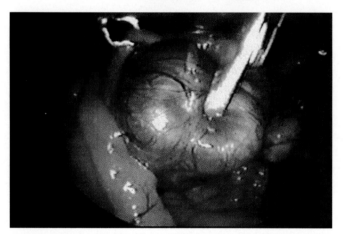

Figure 6.2a and 6.2b *Incision at the avascular line.*

2. Using laparoscopic scissors, the tube is incised at the centre of the radial scars. These are the sites of fusion of the fimbrial folds (Fig. 6.2). Electrocautery and CO_2 laser may also be used, but are not advocated because of the associated thermal damage.

3. The scissors enter the lumen of the tube through this incision. The blades are opened to retain the scissors within the tube. The grasping forceps are transferred to the edge of the newly created ostium. The blades of the scissors are closed and the grasping forceps and scissors are spread apart to stretch and enlarge the ostium of the tube (Fig. 6.3).

4. Additional radial incisions of the tubal wall open the ostium to its full extent.

5. Three or four microsutures of 6-0 polypropylene are placed with a knot pushed around the ostium to pin back the cut edge of the tube to the ampulla (Figs 6.4, 6.5 and 6.6). Other eversion techniques have been described, for example the "Bruhat" procedure. A defocused laser is applied to the serosa of the distal ampulla so as to cause serosal contraction and (hopefully) eversion of the mucosa. Detractors of this technique point to the inevitable thermal damage to the oviduct.

6. The pelvis is lavaged and several hundred millilitres of lactated Ringer's solution is left in the peritoneal cavity.

Figure 6.3a

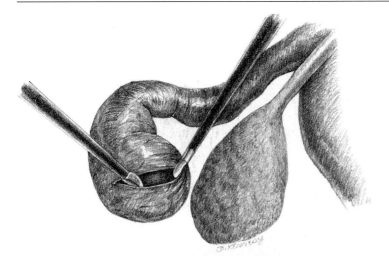

Figure 6.3b

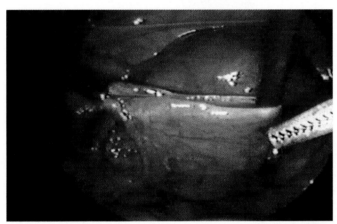

Figure 6.3 and 6.3b *Enlargement of the neo-ostium by stretching the opening.*

FIMBRIAL PHIMOSIS REPAIR

An identical technique is performed as for hydrosalpinx repair. It is notable that the presence of fimbrial tissue on the external surface of a phimotic tube may not be the actual site of the phimotic lumen (Fig. 6.7). Care is taken to pinpoint the lumen by injecting dye solution transcervically. The procedure is as follows.

1. Scissors enter the lumen without incision if possible, or after enlarging the ostium.
2. The ostium is stretched between the scissors and the grasping forceps.
3. Additional radial incisions are placed.
4. The cut edges of the new ostium are sutured to the ampulla with three or four microsutures of 6-0 polypropylene.
5. The pelvis is lavaged and several hundred millilitres of lactated Ringer's solution is left in the peritoneal cavity.

POTENTIAL COMPLICATIONS AND THEIR PREVENTION

1. Haemorrhage by inadvertent incision of the mesosalpinx. This occurs when intratubal chromopertubation fluid leaks from the hydrosalpinx into the mesosalpinx. The interstitium of the mesosalpinx is distended resembling the terminus of the hydrosalpinx. If this is not recognized by the surgeon, the mesosalpinx will be incised. The vascular

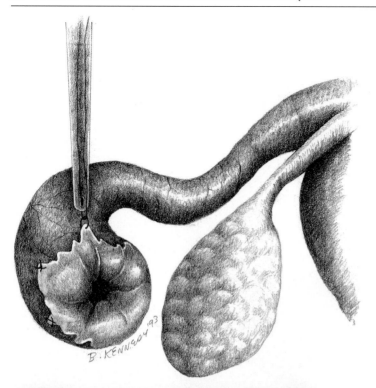

Figure 6.4 *Eversion of the mucosal flap with sutures.*

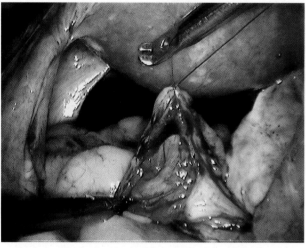

Figure 6.5 *Eversion of the mucosal flap with sutures.*

supply of the mesosalpinx is extensive and the vessels are relatively unsupported. Incision of these vessels can lead to profuse bleeding and haematoma formation.
2. Trauma to the tubal tissues. Excessive handling of the tube and the use of thermal energies such as laser and electrocautery may lead to scarring and tubal reocclusion. Sharp dissection is the least damaging to the tubal mucosa.

CONTRAINDICATIONS

1. In the presence of associated tubal disease proximally, such as salpingitis isthmica nodosa and/or obstruction, distal

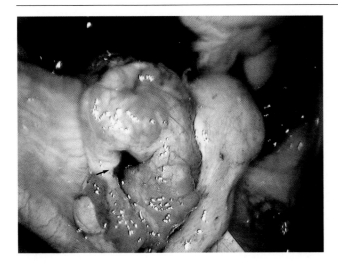

Figure 6.6 *Tubal patency is ascertained by the passage of methylene blue solution* (arrow).

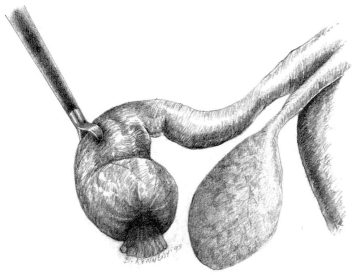

Figure 6.7 *Fimbrial tissue lateral to the phimotic ostium.*

neosalpingostomy rarely results in fertility, even when the proximal disease has been excised. Repair of bipolar tubal blockage (proximal and distal occlusion) rarely results in fertility other than ectopic pregnancy.

2. The presence of honeycomb loculated adhesions within the lumen of the tube not only precludes adequate eversion of the mucosa at salpingostomy but is predictive of poor subsequent fertility. These adhesions may be identified by a "leopard skin" appearance of the ampullary image at hysterosalpingography before the laparoscopy.

SUGGESTED READING

Boer-Meisel ME, Te Velde ER, Habbema JDF, Kardaun JWPF: Predicting the pregnancy outcome in patients treated for hydrosalpinx: a prospective study. *Fertil Steril* 1986 **45**:23–29.

McComb, P: Advances in infertility surgery: can laparoscopy replace microsurgical laparotomy? in Diamond M, (ed) *Infertility Surgery*. Elsevier, New York [*Clinical Practice of Gynecology* 1991 **3**: 1–20].

7

ANASTOMOSIS OF THE FALLOPIAN TUBE

Charles H. Koh

Laparoscopic microsurgery is a technique that combines the potential of conventional microsurgery and laparoscopy. It can overcome the deficits inherent in each. There are concerns that crude macrosurgical laparoscopic surgery may cause irreparable tissue damage which are possibly avoidable by conventional open microsurgery. These concerns are legitimate and are addressed by this new tool. In fact as our experience and technique of laparoscopic microsurgery has evolved and improved, it is becoming evident that we are exceeding our surgical expectations, moving beyond "new access, old technique" into the era of what we would call "new access, new technique". This is the technique of "continuous microsurgery" only achievable via laparoscopy.

Reproductive surgery can now be performed in ways that neither operative laparoscopy nor conventional microsurgery were able to.

INDICATIONS

1. Reversal of sterilization.
2. Mid-tubal blockage secondary to pathology.
3. Tubal occlusion after treatment of ectopic pregnancy.
4. Salpingitis isthmica nodosa.
5. Failed tubal cannulation for proximal blockage.
6. Failed previous macrosurgical sterilization reversal.

EQUIPMENT AND INSTRUMENTS

Magnification, resolution, digital enhancement.

Magnification of 25–40 times is essential to identify healthy mucosa and muscularis before anastomosis can be performed. For microsuturing, magnification at 10–15 times is adequate. We measure laparoscopic magnification by using a 20 inch monitor and determining the ratio of the size of the image on the monitor to actual life size. We call it the "magnification factor of video laparoscopy". With the current three-chip cameras available with zoom capability, magnification up to 40× is achievable.

Magnification requires a corresponding high resolution to be usable, and this is achieved by cameras and monitors capable of 800 lines of resolution. The three-chip camera is also indispensable for accurate colour resolution. An 8-0 suture which is 45 μm in diameter is easily seen using such a video system. To further enhance contrast, some companies have built-in digital enhancement in their cameras or as an add-on unit. This enhances small vessels and edge detail thus improving discrimination. Extremely sensitive auto-iris built into the camera provides rapid control of illumination, avoiding the dreaded "white-out" when the telescope is brought close to tissue. This is particularly important in microsuturing as the telescope has to be panned in and out frequently during the case.

Microinstrumentation

We have designed microinstrumentation that allows laparoscopic microsuturing with precision and ease. This avoids the inefficiency and frustration caused by suture fraying and breakage and poor needle stability. Special design elements include sand-blasted tips to reduce glare, atraumatic terminal serrations, jaw apposition without slippage of 8/0 suture, and a sensitive handle design.

Sutures and needles

A more rigid needle is necessary for laparoscopic microsuturing than for classical microsurgery. Furthermore, it is often easier to insert the needle directly into tissue without the use of a counterpressing grasper. To achieve this the needle needs low force penetration characteristics and superior rigidity. Suitable examples include the BV 175-6 needle swaged to 7-0 and 8-0 Prolene or a BV 130-5 needle swaged to 8-0 polypropylene (Ethalloy TruTaper needle, Ethicon). Another excellent needle is the Surgipro 135-5 needle swaged to 8-0 polypropylene (US Surgical Corporation). Although black nylon would give better discrimination laparoscopically, the needle is not ideal. Plain Vicryl is the most difficult to see laparoscopically and becomes limp when wet. Monofilament sutures tend not to fray and allow easier intracorporeal suturing.

Other equipment

- Reusable 3-mm trocars are available with the Koh Ultramicro Series, or 5-mm trocars with 3-mm reducers may be used.
- Three mm suction irrigators are available

and provide a more suitable jet for micro-surgery than the 5-mm counterparts.
- Stents are not used as it can be traumatic to cannulate the distal fallopian tube.
- The Rumi uterine manipulator with its superior anteversion mechanism is indispensable for tubal anastomosis as multiple permutations of uterine position can be obtained, thereby presenting the proximal tube at a favourable angle for micro-suturing. The lateral openings of the Rumi intrauterine tip facilitate retrograde chromopertubation. Uterine manipulators with a terminal opening tend to be lodged in the endometrium and cause intravasation of dye and a false diagnosis of a proximal block.
- A $150 \mu m$ microneedle tip unipolar electrode is used for incision and dissection, powered from a low voltage generator. Power settings of 15–20 W for cutting and 15 W for fulguration are adequate. When the mesenteric vasculature is inadvertently cut causing more vigorous bleeding, a microbipolar electrode of 1 mm diameter is used.

PREREQUISITES OF SURGEONS

The aspiring laparoscopic microsurgeon should be highly experienced in classical microsurgery and have highly developed two-handed laparoscopic skills for intracorporeal knotting. Extracorporal techniques for 7-0 and 8-0 sutures are impractical and crude and cause "cutting through" or disruption of tissue.

TYPES OF ANASTOMOSIS

Isthmic–isthmic anastomosis

Although the lumen may be as small as $500 \mu m$ to 1 mm, equivalent luminal size and a thick muscularis allows a technically easier anastomosis, particularly if 8-0 suture is used.

Isthmic–ampullary anastomosis

In this case luminal disparity is a potential problem. Preliminary dissection of the serosa and visualization of the proximal stump makes it possible to create a lumen only slightly larger than the proximal ostium.

Ampullary–ampullary anastomosis

The awkwardness in these cases is due to the thin muscularis and the tendency for prolapse or extrusion of the mucosal folds. The angled probe can be used to delineate the muscularis and to push the redundant mucosa back into the lumen after tying the muscularis sutures.

Tubal–cornual anastomosis

A linear slit at the 12 o'clock position is made in the cornual muscularis, using the microneedle electrode after pitressin injection. This allows some mobility of the interstitial tube so that it can be aligned to the needle and needle holder to effect suturing.

SELECTION OF CASES FOR BEGINNERS

The easier cases to perform laparoscopic microsurgical anastomosis are mechanical sterilizations. The tissue damage is predictable and there is enough proximal and distal tube available. In particular, the availability of proximal tube allows its mobilization to conform with the needle position. With cornual anastomosis, extra steps are needed to mobilize the intramural tube and the suture placement may be inaccurate without a considerable amount of experience. Therefore, cases of electrosurgical sterilization, salpingitis isthmica nodosa and failed tubal cannulation are not suitable for anastomosis until the operator has performed more than 50 cases of mid-tubal anastomosis with good outcome. In this regard, a preoperative hysterosalpingogram may provide good prescreening.

PROCEDURE

1. After insertion of a Foley catheter, a uterine manipulator with appropriate tip is inserted into the uterus for mobilization. The intrauterine balloon is inflated with 3 ml of saline. Dilute methylene blue is attached via syringe to the chromopertubation port. We employ the direct puncture technique using a 10-mm disposable trocar through the umbilical incision. After pneumoperitoneum has been created under direct visualization the secondary ports are then placed (3 or 5 mm with reducer). The uterus is then mobilized and anteverted and retroverted to inspect the pelvis. The length of the proximal and distal tube are examined and the condition of the fimbria evaluated. Any paratubal and periovarian adhesions are first removed, using the microelectrode. If all conditions are satisfactory for anastomosis, the operation proceeds.

2. The pitressin injector is inserted through the right lower port and 1:30 dilute pitressin is injected into the terminal serosa of the proximal tube – just enough to bulge the serosa. Next, using the ultra-micro-I grasper with the left hand to stabilize the tip of the tube, the operator introduces the microneedle electrode through the right lower port to circumscribe the serosa of the proximal tube about 5 mm from the tip. If the tubal length is generous and there is obvious bulbous dilatation of the tip, more tube can be sacrificed and the serosal cut would be 1 cm away from the tip. Then, the microneedle is used to divide the tubal mesentery up to the chosen point for transection. By keeping this incision close to the tube, the mesosalpingeal vessels are not damaged and, therefore, do not require cautery, which may compromise the blood supply to the fallopian tube.

3. The guillotine is inserted into the right lower port and a right-angled cut is made of the proximal tube. Chromopertubation

is performed retrogradely by means of the syringe attached to the uterine manipulator. When dye emerges freely from the proximal tube, the laparoscope is brought to within 1 cm of the tissue to examine the muscularis and the mucosa at 40× magnification (Fig. 7.1). Normal isthmic mucosa stains blue and exhibits three or four folds. The muscularis is found to be circular and non-fibrotic.

The proximal end of the distal tube is now held up and pitressin is injected subserosally via the right lower port. The microelectrode is then used to dissect and expose the proximal stump of the distal tube, which is regrasped using the Ultramicro II grasper at the very tip. At this point, the tubal lumen is compared to that of the proximal tube by using the straight chromopertubator, which has 1 mm markings along its tip. The aim is to obtain a distal lumen that is no more than 1 mm larger than the proximal stump.

The guillotine is then reintroduced to cut the distal stump. The curved chromopertubator is then introduced to inject methylene blue dye through the proximal lumen gently to see that it emerges through the fimbria. This confirms patency of the distal tube without the need for cannulation, which is more difficult to achieve laparoscopically and trau-

matic. The lumen is inspected to ensure that the size is adequate and if not, further cuts are made with the guillotine. Pinpoint haemostasis is performed as necessary. Any redundant segment of fallopian tube with attached loop or clip may now be removed using the unipolar electrode.

4. An 8-cm length of 6-0 nylon or Prolene is now introduced by holding the suture 2 cm from the needle. This is introduced using the ultramicro-I through the right upper quadrant with the operator's left hand. The needle holder in the operator's right hand is introduced into the right lower quadrant (Fig. 7.2). The needle is grasped by the needle holder and positioned with the help of the grasper. The mesosalpinx is sutured together using intracorporal knot tying about 5 mm away from the fallopian tube. Care should be taken not to approximate the mesosalpinx too near the tube as it will hinder subsequent anastomosis.

5. A 6 cm length of 7-0 or 8-0 suture is now introduced in the same way as previously and the needle is positioned similarly on the needle holder. Using clockwise rotation of the wrist, the muscularis at 6 o'clock on the distal tube is pierced, avoiding the mucosa. The needle is then inserted at 6 o'clock of the proximal tube

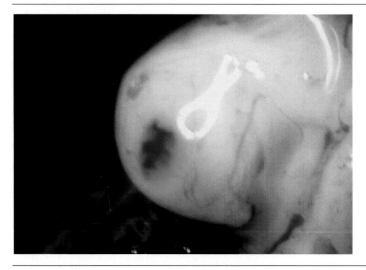

Figure 7.1 *Midtubal anastomosis: the proximal tubal stump has been cut revealing normal mucosa and patency.*

from submucosa through muscularis, again maintaining the clockwise motion of the wrist. Intracorporal knot tying is performed with three knots thrown. This is then cut, using the suture scissors.

Another 7-0 or 8-0 suture is placed at 12 o'clock of the proximal tube from muscularis to submucosa and then to the 12 o'clock position of the distal tube with the needle entering from submucosa through muscularis (Fig. 7.3). This suture is now held by the assistant and together with the use of the uterine manipulator, one is able to rotate the tube so that both the 3 and 9 o'clock positions become available for accurate suture placement. These are placed next and tied and finally, the 12 o'clock suture is tied (Figs 7.4–7.10). Chromopertubation is performed via the uterine manipulator and patency of the tube can now be demonstrated. Slight leakage at the anastomotic site is no cause for concern as long as dye emerges from the distal fimbria. 6-0 Prolene or nylon is then used to place two or three interrupted serosal sutures. These sutures should also incorporate the outer muscularis to maintain strength of the anastomosis. Any gaps evident in the mesosalpinx are similarly closed using 6-0 nylon (Fig. 7.11). The opposite tube is then treated in the same manner.

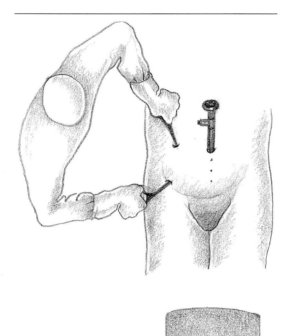

Figure 7.2 *The position of the surgeon.*

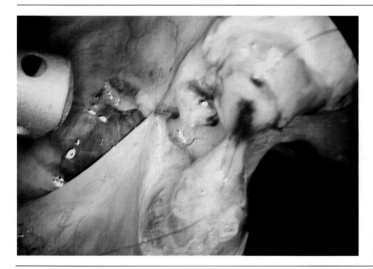

Figure 7.3 *The six o'clock suture has been tied. The 12 o'clock suture is placed.*

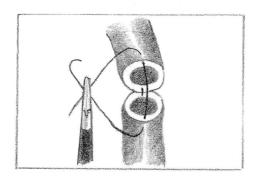

Figure 7.4 *The 12 o'clock suture is held.*

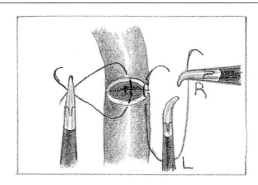

Figure 7.5

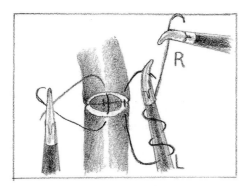

Figure 7.6

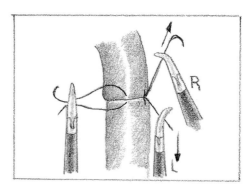

Figure 7.7

Figures 7.5–7.7 *Rotation of the 12 o'clock suture to the opposite side allows the 3 o'clock suture to be placed and tied.*

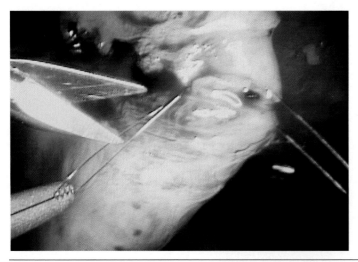

Figure 7.8 *The 12 o'clock suture is moved to allow the 9 o'clock suture to be placed and tied.*

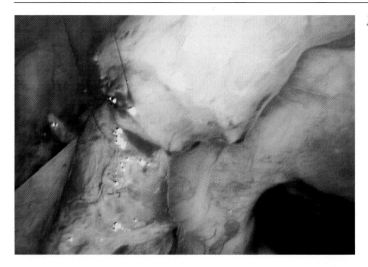

Figure 7.9

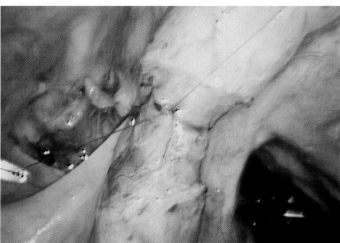

Figure 7.10

Figures 7.9–7.10 *The 12 o'clock
suture is tied.*

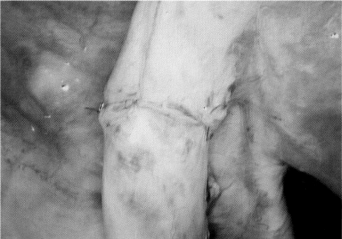

Figure 7.11 *Anastomosis is
completed.*

CONCLUSIONS

Laparoscopic microsurgery is an exciting new tool with great potential beyond classical microsurgery. However, the learning curve is steep and skill development is very intensive. It requires at least 20 midtubal cases before operators begin to develop a fluid rhythm. After 50 cases one can perform bilateral midtubal anastomosis in 90 minutes, making it a very efficient procedure.

SUGGESTED READING

Brosens IA: Risks and benefits of endoscopic surgery in reproductive medicine. *Proceedings of the 15th World Congress of Fertility and Sterility* 1995 **47**: 339–343.

Koh CH, Janik GM: Laparoscopic microsurgical tubal anastomosis. In Adamson GD and Martin DC (eds) *Endoscopic Management of Gynecologic Diseases*. Lippincott, Raven Press, Philadelphia, PA, 1996, vol. 13, pp. 119–145.

8

TUBAL ECTOPIC PREGNANCY: SALPINGOSTOMY AND SALPINGECTOMY

Togas Tulandi

SALPINGOSTOMY

Despite an increasing popularity of methotrexate treatment, surgical management remains the most definite and universal treatment of ectopic pregnancy. Contrary to surgical treatment, tubal rupture can still occur after methotrexate treatment. The procedure requires three laparoscopic punctures including a 10-mm puncture for easy removal of the specimen. Because of the possibility of encountering haemoperitoneum, the laparoscope should be inserted into the peritoneal cavity gradually (Fig. 8.1), otherwise the lens will be stained with blood and it could be a nuisance.

The presence of haemoperitoneum should not prevent laparoscopic treatment of ectopic pregnancy. Using a suction irrigator, the blood can be evacuated and the pelvic organs are irrigated with physiological saline or Ringer's lactate solution. Careful inspection should be done and the ectopic pregnancy is identified (Fig. 8.2). The tube is then immobilized with laparoscopy forceps. Using a 22-gauge injection needle inserted through a 5-mm portal, a solution of vasopressin (0.2 IU/ml of

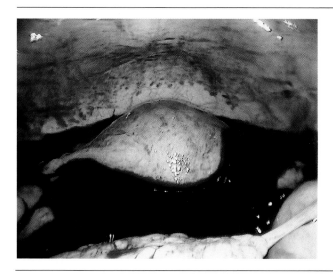

Figure 8.1 Because of the possibility of encountering haemoperitoneum, the laparoscope should be inserted into the peritoneal cavity gradually.

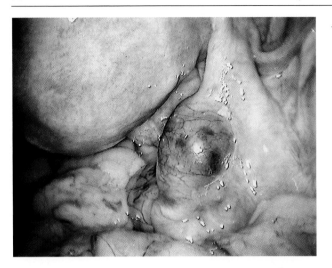

Figure 8.2 *A right ampullary pregnancy.*

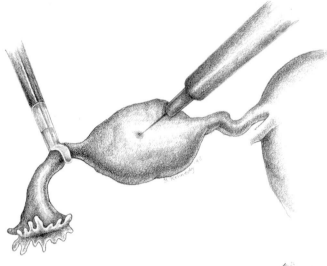

Figure 8.3 *Linear salpingostomy: injection of vasopressin into the wall of the tube.*

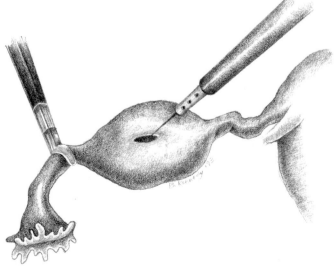

Figure 8.4 *A longitudinal incision is made on the antemesosalpinx of the tube.*

physiological saline) is injected into the wall of the tube at the area of maximal distention (Fig. 8.3). This will allow surgery with minimal bleeding. A 10–15-mm longitudinal incision is made on the maximally distended antemesosalpinx wall of the tube. Either laser with power density of 10 000 W/cm^2 for a CO_2 laser, unipolar needle electrocautery (cutting current of 10 W) or scissors can be used (Fig. 8.4). The products of conception (Fig. 8.5) are flushed out of the tube with high-pressure irrigating solution. Using a combination of hydrodissection and gentle blunt dissection with a suction irriga-tor, the products of conception are removed from the tube (Fig. 8.6). This technique is preferable to piecemeal removal with forceps. The specimen is removed with a 10-mm claw forceps or placed in an endoscopic bag. An endoscopic bag that automatically opens in the abdominal cavity (Rx Endo-catch, Autosuture, Norwalk, Connecticut) is preferable. It can be difficult and time consuming to open a rolled endoscopic bag. The specimen is then removed from the abdominal cavity (Figs 8.7a and 8.7b).

The tube is carefully irrigated and inspected "under water" for haemostasis.

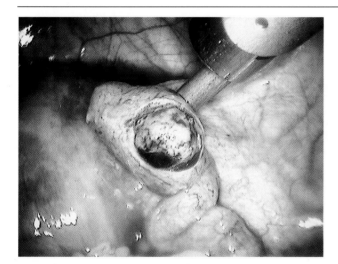

Figure 8.5 *The products of conception are seen inside the tube. Note the vasopressin-blanching effects on the tissue.*

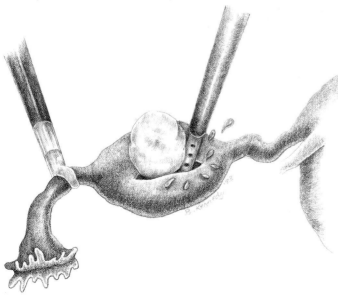

Figure 8.6 *By using a suction irrigator, the products of conception are flushed out of the tube.*

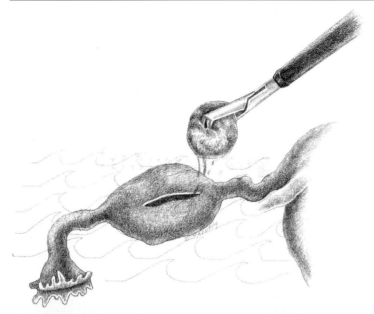

Figure 8.7a

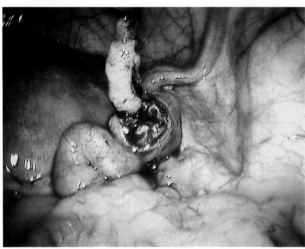

Figure 8.7b

Figures 8.7a and 8.7b *Removal of the products of conception using a claw forceps.*

Bleeding points can be coagulated with micro-bipolar forceps. Persistent bleeding from the "placental bed" can be controlled by placing a suture ligature with 6-0 Vicryl in the mesosalpinx (Fig. 8.8). The tubal incision is left open to heal by secondary intention. Before terminating the procedure, approximately 500–1000 ml of Ringer's lactate solution is left in the abdominal cavity and the pelvic organs once again inspected for accurate haemostasis ("examination under water").

SALPINGECTOMY

Salpingectomy with electrocautery

In the presence of persistent bleeding or ruptured tubal pregnancy, a salpingectomy is an alternative. Obviously, if the patient is unstable, an immediate laparotomy should be done. The tube is immobilized with a grasping forceps. The tubal segment to be excised is coagulated with a bipolar cautery and cut (Figs 8.9 and 8.10). The procedure is repeated on the mesosalpinx of the tubal segment to be excised and on the distal

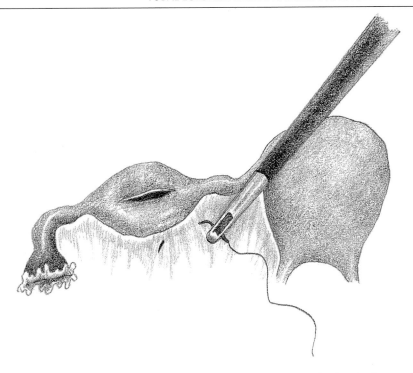

Figure 8.8 *Suturing the vessels in the mesosalpinx using 6-0 polyglactin for persistent bleeding.*

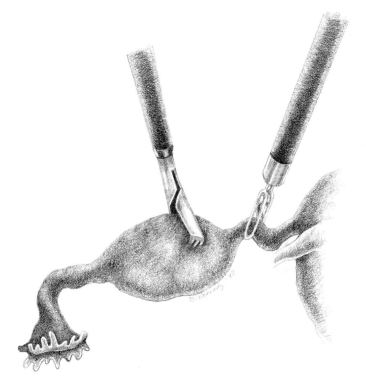

Figure 8.9 *Salpingectomy with electrocautery: coagulation of the tubal segment that will be removed.*

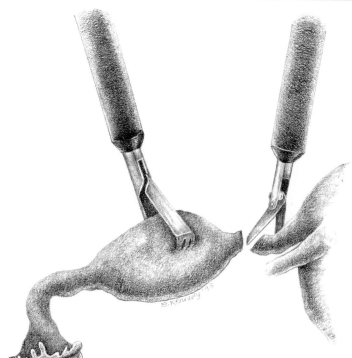

Figure 8.10 *Cutting of the coagulated tube.*

Figure 8.11

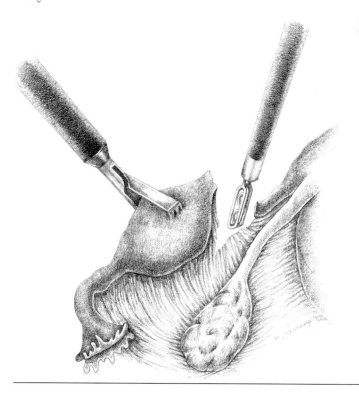

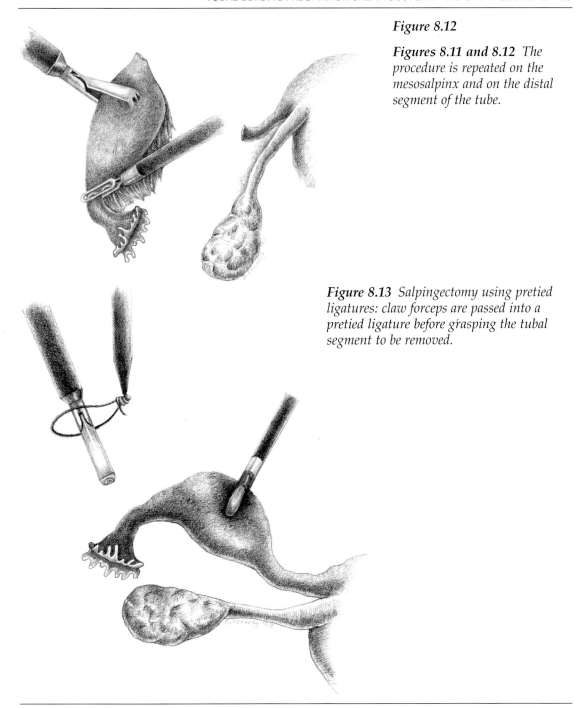

Figure 8.12

Figures 8.11 and 8.12 *The procedure is repeated on the mesosalpinx and on the distal segment of the tube.*

Figure 8.13 *Salpingectomy using pretied ligatures: claw forceps are passed into a pretied ligature before grasping the tubal segment to be removed.*

portion of the tube (Figs 8.11 and 8.12). Unipolar scissors can also be used for simultaneous coagulation and cutting. Large vessels, however, have to be coagulated with bipolar forceps. Partial salpingectomy or distal salpingectomy can be done. The tube is removed and careful haemostasis is done as described above. The procedure has also been used for cornual pregnancies.

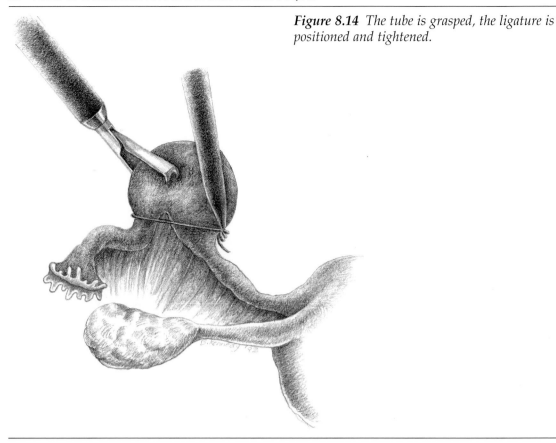

Figure 8.14 *The tube is grasped, the ligature is positioned and tightened.*

Salpingectomy with a pretied ligature (Endoloop, PercLoop)

Salpingectomy can also be done using a pretied ligature (Endoloop, Rx Ethicon Inc., Sommerville, NJ; PercLoop, Laparomed, Irvine, CA). The loop is first inserted into the abdominal cavity. A grasping forceps is passed into the loop and the tube is grasped (Fig. 8.13). The portion of the tube that contains an ectopic pregnancy is lifted and a loop is placed at the base and tightened (Fig. 8.14). Another loop is placed above the first. The tubal segment is then cut above the loops (Fig. 8.15). If the pedicle is too large, the loop might slip. Salpingectomy with electrocautery is a preferred method.

COMPLICATIONS AND THEIR PREVENTION

The possibility of leaving products of conception by laparoscopy is similar to that by laparotomy (up to 5%). To avoid this complication, careful attention should be given to the medial portion of the tube. This is the area where the trophoblastic tissue can be inadvertently left behind causing persistent elevation of serum human chorionic gonadotrophin levels postoperatively. In this situation, a single dose of methotrexate administration (1 mg/kg body weight, intramuscularly) will usually solve the problem.

CONTRAINDICATIONS

Patients who are haemodynamically unstable should undergo an immediate laparotomy.

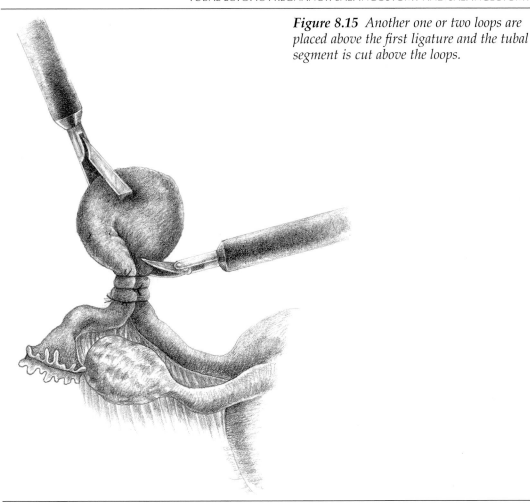

Figure 8.15 *Another one or two loops are placed above the first ligature and the tubal segment is cut above the loops.*

SUGGESTED READING

Lundorff P, Thorburn J, Lindblom B: Fertility outcome after conservative surgical treatment of ectopic pregnancy evaluated in a randomized trial. *Fertil Steril* 1992 **57**: 998–1002.

Pouly JL, Mahnes H, Mage G, Canis M, Bruhat MA: Conservative laparoscopic treatment of 321 ectopic pregnancies. *Fertil Steril* 1986 **46**: 1093–1097.

Tulandi T, Vilos G, Gomel V: Laparoscopic treatment of cornual pregnancy. *Obstet Gynecol* 1995 **85**: 465–467.

Yao M, Tulandi T: Current status of surgical and non-surgical treatment of ectopic pregnancy. *Fertil Steril* 1997 **67**: 421–433.

9

OVARIAN CYSTECTOMY

Togas Tulandi

OVARIAN CYSTECTOMY

Ovarian cysts in premenopausal women are rarely malignant and ovarian cystectomy can be done safely. The incidence of malignancy is approximately 0.4%. It is lower in younger women and in those with a unilocular cyst. A preoperative transvaginal ultrasonogram is beneficial to evaluate the type of tumour. The diagnosis is usually accurate for an endometrioma or a dermoid cyst. Serum CA-125 has been used as a marker for epithelial ovarian carcinoma, but in premenopausal women, it has poor sensitivity and specificity.

For ovarian cystectomy, one of the secondary trocars should be at least 10 mm for removal of the specimen. The whole abdominal cavity including the liver and diaphragm should be first thoroughly evaluated. Suspicious lesions should be biopsied and sent for frozen section examination. Peritoneal fluid is sent for cytology. The ovarian cyst is exposed by elevating it with a forceps behind the ovary or by grasping the utero-ovarian ligament (Fig. 9.1). Sometimes, it is necessary for lysis of adhesions to be performed first.

The cyst is palpated with a laparoscopic probe or forceps. Using a 22-gauge injection needle inserted through a secondary portal, 5–10 ml of physiological saline is injected into the ovarian capsule (Figs 9.2a and 9.2b). This creates a cleavage plane by separating

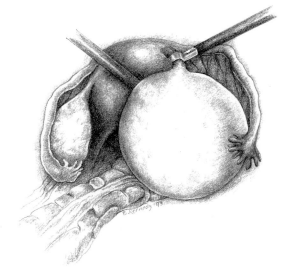

Figure 9.1 *The ovarian cyst is exposed by elevating it with a forceps behind the ovary or by grasping the utero-ovarian ligament.*

the capsule from the cyst wall. A spinal needle can be used also. This is inserted transcutaneously, but it bends easily and is more difficult to manipulate. A superficial incision is made on the ovarian capsule with scissors without entering the cyst (Fig. 9.3).

Using a combination of hydrodissection and blunt dissection with a suction irrigator, the cleavage plane is further developed. This is usually easy to achieve especially with a dermoid cyst but not with an

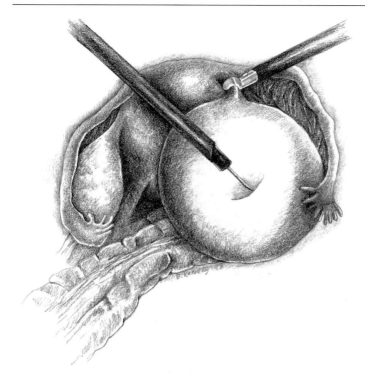

Figure 9.2a

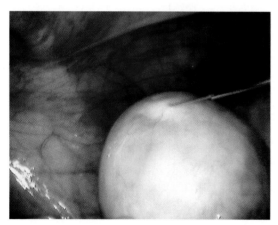

Figure 9.2b

Figures 9.2a and 9.2b *Creating a cleavage plane by injecting physiological saline into the ovarian capsule.*

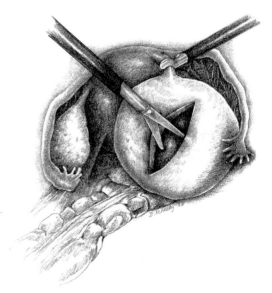

Figure 9.3 *A superficial incision is made on the ovarian capsule without entering the cyst.*

endometriotic cyst. Hydrodissection is done using physiological saline or Ringer's lactate solution (Figs 9.4 and 9.5). The capsule is held by laparoscopic forceps and the unruptured cyst can be enucleated entirely (Fig. 9.6).

If there is concern of intraperitoneal spillage of malignant cells, the ovarian cyst is better removed intact and puncture should be avoided. The unruptured cyst is

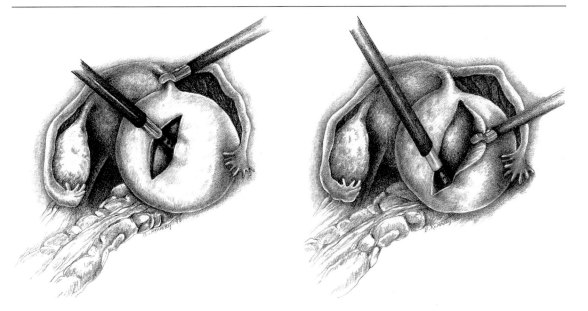

Figure 9.4

Figure 9.5

Figure 9.6a

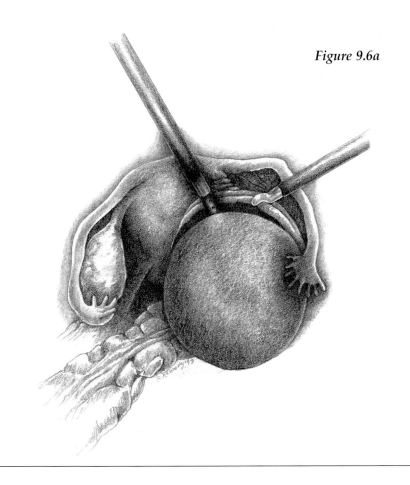

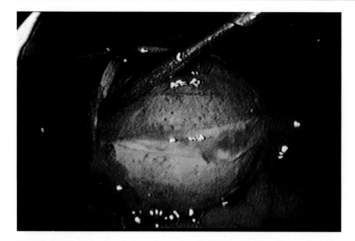

Figure 9.6b

Figures 9.4, 9.5, 9.6a and 9.6b
Enucleation of the cyst using hydrodissection.

placed in a laparoscopic pouch inserted via a 10-mm secondary trocar. There are several types of laparoscopic pouch available. The most practical is a pouch that opens automatically after insertion into the abdominal cavity (Rx Endocatch, Autosuture, Norwalk, Connecticut). The specimen can be inserted into the pouch with ease. Other types have to be opened in the abdominal cavity and this may take time. The pouch is then retracted from the abdominal cavity and the trocar is removed. The pouch is held tight against the abdominal wall and is opened (Fig. 9.7). The cyst wall seen just under the abdominal wall is incised using a regular scalpel, a suction irrigator is immediately inserted into the cyst and the cyst contents are aspirated. Once the cyst collapses, the pouch with the cyst wall inside slides out of the abdominal cavity. Sometimes the cyst's contents are very thick and the cyst has to be irrigated repeatedly with solution of Ringer's lactate. In the case of dermoid cyst, the hair and sometimes tooth or bones can be extracted using Kelly forceps inside the pouch. Not uncommonly, a portion of the cyst can be delivered out of the abdomen, but the bulk of the cyst remains inside the abdomen. Here the extracorporeal site of the cyst is opened and the contents removed. With the techniques described, not only is intraperitoneal spillage avoided, but also the potential of implanting possible cancer cells in the trocar site is eliminated.

Care should be taken so as not to spill the contents of the cyst during surgery. However, endometriomas tend to have a thin wall and spillage often occurs. This does not seem to be associated with adverse outcome. We have also found similar findings after spillage of the contents of dermoid

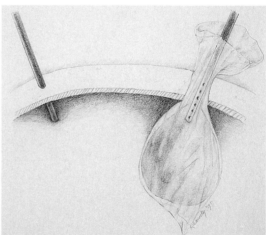

Figure 9.7 *The endoscopic pouch is held tight against the abdominal wall and opened and the contents of the cyst are aspirated. From Tulandi T: Difficulties of removing specimen from the abdominal cavity at laparoscopy. In Corfman R, Diamond MP, De Cherney AH (eds) Complications of Laparoscopy and Hysteroscopy. Blackwell Science, Oxford, 1997. Reprinted by permission.*

cyst. This is due to extensive irrigation of the peritoneal cavity at the completion of the procedure. It also appears that spillage of the contents of benign mucinous cysts does not cause pseudomyxoma peritonei. However, spillage should be avoided as far as possible.

Sometimes the cyst inadvertently ruptures during the dissection. In this situation, the contents are aspirated and the cyst is repeatedly irrigated with physiological saline until clean. The inner surface of the cyst is carefully inspected for possible malignancy. If vegetations are found, examination of a frozen section is immediately performed. The findings of cancer cells should be followed by immediate laparotomy for staging and treatment. Otherwise, a laparoscopic ovarian cystectomy or oophorectomy is done. If frozen section is not available, it is better to wait for histopathological confirmation. The decision is based on the patient's menopausal status and clinically. Several studies have suggested that the prognosis is not influenced by spillage of a malignant tumour if immediate treatment is given. Other studies suggest that intraoperative spillage of a malignant tumour may worsen the prognosis. Certainly, the prognosis is impaired if the treatment is delayed for several weeks.

In the absence of suspicious lesions, ovarian cystectomy is done by stripping the cyst wall from the ovarian tissue. The cyst wall is grasped with toothed forceps for traction and dissection. This is facilitated by grasping the cyst wall and the ovarian tissue with two forceps close to each other for traction and countertraction (Figs 9.8–9.10). Sometimes, blood vessels at the base of the cyst are found and these have to be coagulated and divided before the final separation of the cyst wall from the ovary.

Intermittent irrigation of the ovary allows good visualization and helps with accurate haemostasis. Usually, the ovarian defect collapses. However, if the ovary is gaping, two or three sutures of Vicryl 5-0 or tissue sealant can be used to approximate the edges of the ovarian tissue (Fig. 9.11). The ovarian capsule can also be inverted by coagulating the inner side of the ovarian opening (Fig. 9.12). Inversion of the ovarian capsule approximates the ovarian opening. Because of the concerns of coagulating the ovarian blood supply and the normal ovarian tissue leading to premature ovarian failure, this technique is rarely used.

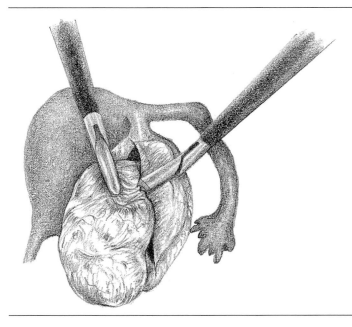

Figure 9.8 *A collapsed cyst wall is grasped with two forceps close to each other for traction and counter-traction.*

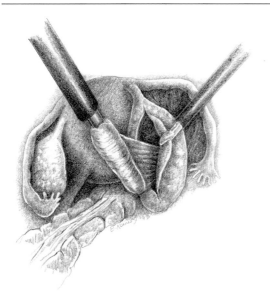

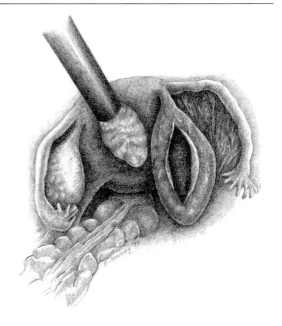

Figure 9.9 *Further separation of the cyst wall using a "hair curler technique".*

Figure 9.10 *Removal of the specimen via a 10-mm secondary portal.*

Figure 9.11 *Three sutures approximating the ovarian opening.*

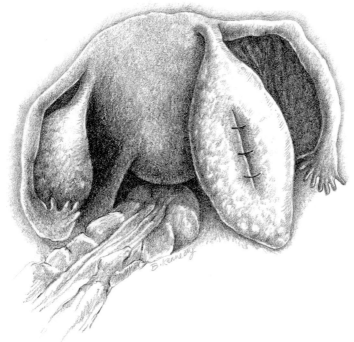

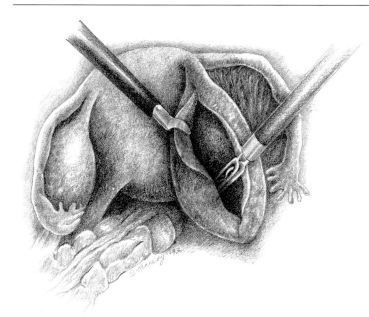

Figure 9.12 *Inversion of the ovarian opening using electrocoagulation.*

Ovarian cysts tend to be bilateral, therefore it is important to examine the opposite ovary. Although, some surgeons remove specimens via an enlarged subumbilical incision, removal via the site of a secondary trocar is preferable. Here, removal is done under direct laparoscopic control. If the specimen is dropped, it will be immediately seen and can be grasped again. Another alternative is to deliver the specimen into the vagina via a posterior colpotomy incision. Colpotomy is done by incising the vagina transversely with a laser or with a unipolar needle electrode. The posterior fornix is pushed upward using a wet sponge at the end of a ring forceps inside the vagina and behind the cervix. The incision is made transversely on the bulging vagina. The location of the rectum should be noted to avoid cutting it. Occasionally, a rectal probe is also required to ascertain that the rectum is free. The wet sponge inside the vagina prevents loss of pneumoperitoneum. If the cyst cannot be removed intact, the contents of the cyst are drained through the vagina and the cyst is then removed. The colpotomy incision can be closed vaginally or laparoscopically with 2-0 polyglactin (Vicryl). Because of the possible contamina-tion with vaginal flora, this technique is rarely used. At the end of the procedure, "examination under water" is performed to evaluate haemostasis and approximately 500–1000 ml of Ringer's lactate solution is left in the abdominal cavity.

VAPORIZATION OF OVARIAN CYST WALL

Occasionally, the cyst wall is so intimately adherent to the ovarian tissue that a cleavage plane cannot be created. This is often encountered with ovarian endometrioma. In this case, the contents of the cyst are aspirated and the cyst is repeatedly irrigated. The top of the cyst, including the associated "ovarian capsule", is excised (Fig. 9.13). Care should be taken not to remove excessive ovarian tissue. After ascertaining that there is no suspicious lesion, the inner surface of the cyst wall is vaporized either with laser or electrocoagulation. The ovarian tissue can be left open or closed as described above. Because of the possibility of leaving some cyst wall, this technique should be rarely used. Also, normal ovarian tissue and ovarian blood supply can be compromised.

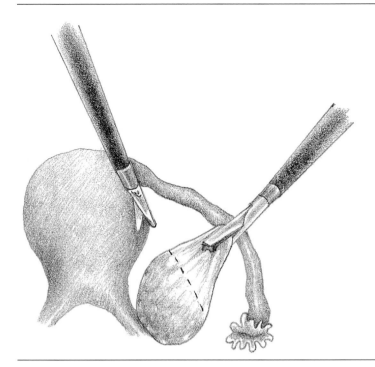

Figure 9.13 *Sometimes the wall of an endometrioma is so intimately adherent to the ovarian tissue and a cleavage plane cannot be created. Here, the top of the cyst including the associated "ovarian capsule" is excised and the inner surface of the cyst wall is vaporized either with laser or electrocoagulation.*

POTENTIAL COMPLICATIONS AND THEIR PREVENTION

1. The possibility of operating on an ovarian malignancy and spilling cancer cells into the peritoneal cavity can be avoided by proper selection of patients before surgery and by careful inspection at the time of laparoscopy. Peritoneal lavage and frozen section should be done for suspicious lesions.
2. Blood vessels especially at the base of the cyst should be coagulated. Although, it is rarely encountered, uncontrollable bleeding requires an immediate laparotomy.
3. Persistent oozing from the inner surface of the ovary after stripping the cyst wall can lead to haematoma formation. A thorough irrigation and haemostasis are mandatory.
4. Potential problems due to spillage of the contents of endometrioma, mucinous cystadenoma or dermoid cyst can be eliminated by liberal irrigation of the peritoneal cavity. It is not uncommon to use 4–5 l of irrigating solution.
5. Another potential complication of ovarian cystectomy is adhesion formation. Meticulous technique, use of non-reactive sutures (not cat-gut) and instillation of a large amount of Ringer's lactate solution might decrease adhesion formation.

CONTRAINDICATIONS

1. Postmenopausal women with a multilocular ovarian cyst are better managed by oophorectomy.
2. Operative laparoscopy is contraindicated if findings of possible ovarian cancer are found preoperatively or at the time of laparoscopy examination.

SUGGESTED READING

Audebert AJM: Laparoscopic ovarian surgery and ovarian torsion. In Sutton C and Diamond M (eds) *Endoscopic Surgery for Gynaecologists*. W.B. Saunders, London, 1993, pp. 134–141.

Nezhat C, Nezhat F, Welander CE, Benigno B: Four ovarian cancers diagnosed during laparoscopic management of 1011 adnexal masses. *Am J Obstet Gynecol* 1992 **167:** 790–796.

Sainz de la Cuesta R, Goff BA, Fuller AF, Nikrui N, Eichhorn JH, Rice LW: Prognostic importance of intraoperative rupture of malignant ovarian epithelial neoplasms. *Obstet Gynecol* 1994 **84**: 1–7.

Tulandi T: Laparoscopy management of ovarian cyst in perimenopausal women. *Gynaecol Endosc* 1996 **5**: 1–4.

10

OOPHORECTOMY AND LARAROSCOPIC ORCHIECTOMY

Togas Tulandi

Removal of the entire ovary especially in postmenopausal women is sometimes indicated. Ovarian cysts in postmenopausal women or persistent pelvic pain due to ovarian endometriosis or periovarian adhesions are possible indications for oophorectomy. Although, it is controversial, women whose first-degree relatives have ovarian cancer and those with breast cancer may also benefit from bilateral oophorectomy. In the presence of an ovarian cyst, preoperative transvaginal ultrasonography and measurement of serum CA 125 are indicated in postmenopausal women.

OOPHORECTOMY

In the presence of an ovarian cyst, a thorough evaluation of the abdominal cavity, peritoneal cytology and examination of frozen section of suspicious lesions should be done as described in Chapter 9. Using grasping forceps inserted through a secondary trocar, the ovary is grasped and pulled medially to expose the mesovarium. Using bipolar cautery, the utero-ovarian ligament is coagulated (Fig. 10.1) and divided. The same procedure is repeated on the mesovarium (Fig. 10.2) until the ovary is

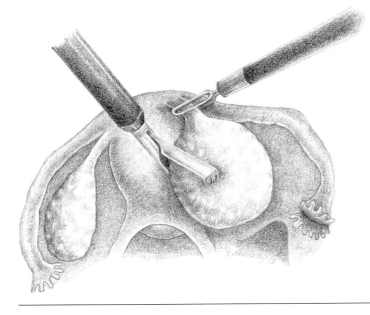

Figure 10.1 Oophorectomy: coagulating the utero-ovarian ligament with bipolar forceps.

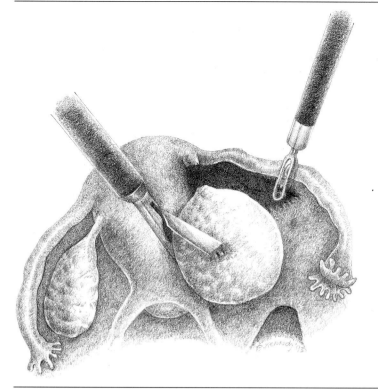

Figure 10.2 *The ovary is retracted medially with a claw forceps.*

completely liberated. This step-by-step technique is especially valuable when the ovary cannot be freely mobilized. To increase the mobility of the ovary, the peritoneum of the broad ligament occasionally has to be hydrodissected away from the pelvic side wall. It is mandatory to follow the course of the ureters before commencing dissection. The ureters enter the pelvis by crossing the external iliac vessels close to the bifurcation of the common iliac vessels. In the pelvis, they run inferior and medial to the hypogastric vessels and then course along the lateral side of uterosacral ligaments to enter the base of the cardinal ligaments. Sometimes, the ureters have to be dissected before commencing with oophorectomy.

If the ovary is not large and free, a simpler technique can be performed. The ovary is retracted medially and a pretied ligature (Endoloops, Rx Ethicon Inc., Sommerville, NJ; PercLoop, Laparomed, Irvine, CA) is placed around the mesovarium and the utero-ovarian ligament and tightened (Figs 10.3 and 10.4). Another ligature is placed

above the first and the pedicle is cut with scissors. Because of the tendency to cut the tissue some distance from the ligature, a part of ovarian tissue could be left behind. The coagulation technique is a better technique. The specimen is then removed. If the specimen is too large, it has to be first morcellated or cut into several pieces intra-abdominally or removed via a colpotomy incision.

SALPINGO-OOPHORECTOMY

In women who have completed their family, a salpingo-oophorectomy is an alternative. This is also a procedure for those who also have damaged fallopian tubes. The course of the ureter is first followed. The ovary and the tube are retracted medially to expose the infundibulopelvic ligament. The ligament is electrocoagulated with a bipolar cautery and is divided (Fig. 10.5). For additional security, a pretied ligature can be placed around the pedicle. The mesosalpinx is then coagulated and divided repeatedly until the cornual part of the tube. The proximal part

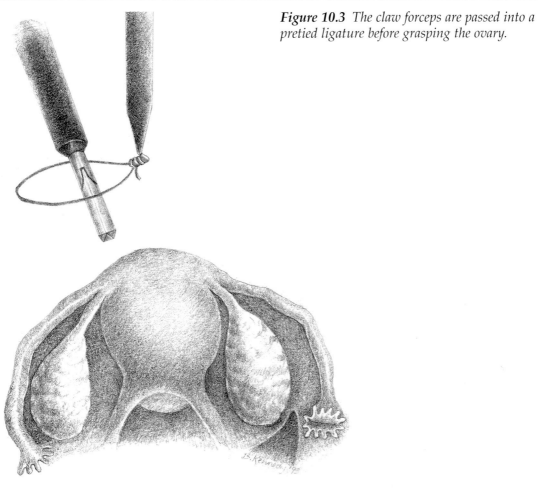

Figure 10.3 *The claw forceps are passed into a pretied ligature before grasping the ovary.*

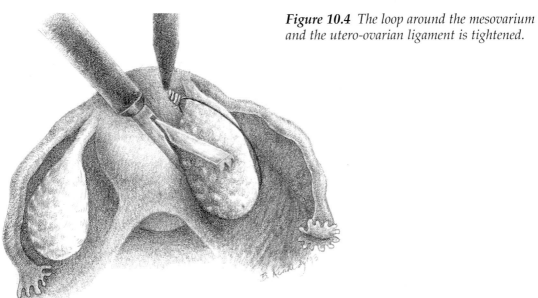

Figure 10.4 *The loop around the mesovarium and the utero-ovarian ligament is tightened.*

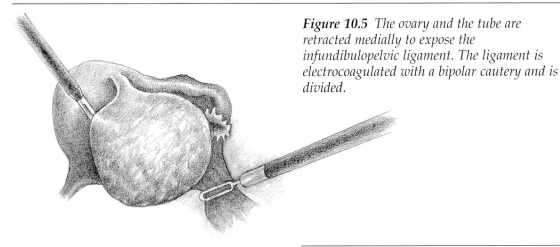

Figure 10.5 *The ovary and the tube are retracted medially to expose the infundibulopelvic ligament. The ligament is electrocoagulated with a bipolar cautery and is divided.*

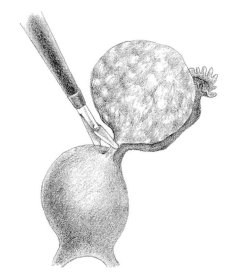

Figure 10.6 *The proximal part of the fallopian tube and the utero-ovarian ligament are treated in the same fashion separating the tube and the ovary from their attachment.*

of the fallopian tube and the utero-ovarian ligament are treated in the same fashion separating the tube and the ovary from their attachment (Fig. 10.6).

LAPAROSCOPIC REMOVAL OF INTRA-ABDOMINAL TESTIS (ORCHIECTOMY)

Although rare, gynecologists can encounter women with androgen insensitivity syn-

drome. The incidence of neoplasia in the intra-abdominal testes in these women is high (about 25%) and the gonads should be removed.

Intra-abdominal testes are usually located between the inguinal ring and the common iliac vessels. The testis is grasped with a grasping forceps and pulled medially (Figs 10.7 and 10.8) . It is gradually and carefully separated from the adjacent peritoneum. The ureters are relatively far from the dissection area, but their course should always be followed.

The plexus pampiniformis that contains the spermatic vessels is skeletonized and two staples are placed on the vessels (Fig. 10.9). This can also be done using bipolar electrocoagulation. The pedicle is then cut below the staples. The adjacent peritoneum on the medial aspect of the testis is cut caudally until the gubernaculum is reached. Two staples are applied on the gubernaculum. It is then divided freeing the testis completely (Fig. 10.10). Pretied ligatures (Endoloop, Percloop) can also be used. The specimen is removed.

COMPLICATIONS AND THEIR PREVENTION

Bleeding and haematoma from the pedicle of the infundibulopelvic ligament can be encountered. Application of a pretied ligature to the coagulated pedicle secures the haemostasis.

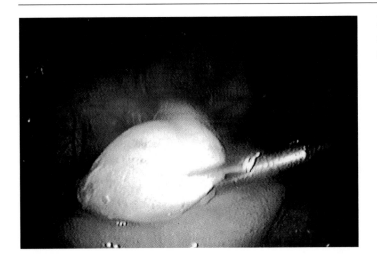

Figure 10.7 Orchiectomy: the left testis is retracted medially with a claw forceps.

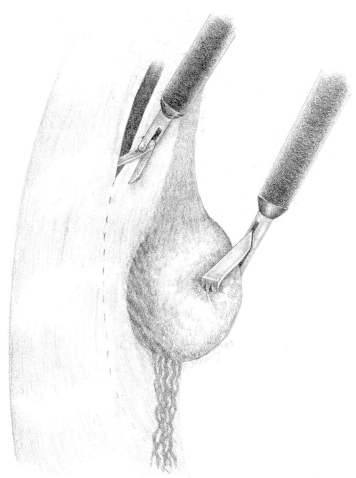

Figure 10.8 Incision of the adjacent peritoneum lateral to the testis with unipolar scissors.

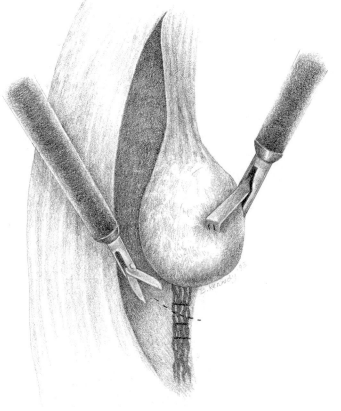

Figure 10.9 *Dividing the plexus pampiniformis between two staples. Plexus pampiniformis is located cranial to the testis.*

Figure 10.10 *The same procedure is done on the gubernaculum.*

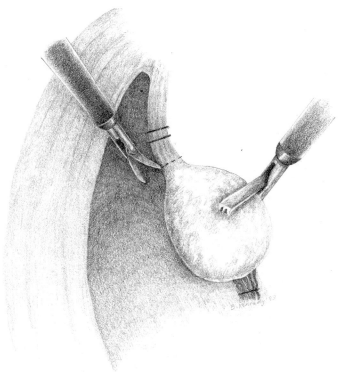

Prevention of ureteral injury should be done by following the course of the ureter before commencing any procedure. During removal of intra-abdominal testes, it is important to know the location of the iliac vessels. Potentially, these major vessels can be injured. Caudally, the bladder can be traumatized.

SUGGESTED READING

Bloom DA, Ayers JWT, McGuire EJ: The role of laparoscopy in the management of nonpalpable testes. *J Urol (Paris)* 1988 **94**: 465.

Daniell JF, Kurtz BR, Lee IY: Laparoscopic oophorectomy: comparative studies of ligatures, bipolar coagulation and automatic stapling devices. *Obstet Gynecol* 1992 **80**: 325–328.

Kristiansen SB, Doody KJ: Laparoscopic removal of 46XY gonads located within the inguinal canals. *Fertil Steril* 1992 **58**: 1076–1077.

Tulandi T, Corcos J, Rochon L: Laparoscopic orchiectomy in a woman with androgen insensitivity syndrome. *J Gynecol Surg* 1994 **10**: 99–101.

11

LAPAROSCOPIC TREATMENT OF ENDOMETRIOSIS

David B. Redwine

Modern conventional treatment of endometriosis has become rigid, unimaginative and dogmatic: laparoscopy with superficial laser vaporization or electrocoagulation of disease, followed by medical therapy, followed by other laparoscopies with more thermal ablation, followed by hysterectomy and castration. The modern view of endometriosis is that it is an enigmatic, chronic, highly recurrent disease which cannot be cured except by hysterectomy and castration. This contrasts sharply with the view of the mid-twentieth century, when Meigs stated that ". . . recurrence is not frequent, and cure of the lesion by conservative surgery is usual." Has the disease changed so much, or are our modern treatments simply less effective than the ancient therapy of cutting the disease out of the body? The answer is obvious – modern therapy is irrational and ineffective. Although laser vaporization has some potential to destroy endometriosis, it frequently does not burn deeply enough to destroy invasive disease. Electrocoagulation of endometriosis has not been described in sufficient detail in the literature to allow surgeons to duplicate its use, and it is universally acknowledged that medical therapy does not eradicate endometriosis of any stage or location. In contrast, laparoscopic excision of endometriosis duplicates the curative potential of excision at laparotomy and can treat disease of any depth or loca-tion without the need for pre- or postoperative medical therapy. The most efficient form of laparoscopic excision is electroexcision, although excision with laser or scissors is possible.

STAGES IN THE PROCEDURE

Safety considerations

Modern monopolar electrosurgery depends on tissue resistance to electron flow generating tissue heat which results in vaporization or coagulation of tissue. Electrons are delivered to the tissue through an active electrode which may be a scissors, needle, grasper, or any other conducting tool. High current density combined with a short dwell time results in a very rapid cutting action with little coagulation effect and essentially no lateral thermal spread. Pure cutting current has a constant but smaller peak to peak voltage than does coagulation current and is primarily used when cutting thin tissue like peritoneum. Coagulation current has a higher peak to peak voltage which provides more power to push electrons through tissue, making coagulation current useful for cutting retroperitoneal fibrosis or parenchymal structures such as the uterosacral ligaments.

In applying electrosurgical energy to tissue, it is necessary to avoid pillowing of tissue around the tip of the active electrode since the greater surface area in contact with tissue will result in a lower current density and increased coagulation effects rather than cutting effects. To avoid undesired pillowing, the electrode is activated before tissue is contacted so cutting begins instantly, and the tissue to be cut is on stretch at all times so that the tissue separates away from the active electrode tip as cutting occurs. The electrode is not always activated, and much of the safety and efficacy of monopolar electrosurgery depends on blunt dissection alternating with brief bursts of electrosurgical cutting when sufficient separation of normal tissue has occurred.

Endometriosis is a disease most commonly found on the peritoneal surface, so excision of involved peritoneum is the fundamental technique used. Whether the surgeon excises endometriosis using scissors, electrosurgery or laser, it is important to separate diseased tissue from normal tissue before application of the surgical energy form. Most commonly this is done by grasping the tissue to be removed and drawing it strongly medially, thus elevating the tissue from underlying vital structures before cutting mechanically, electrosurgically or with a laser. This medial traction is also important to avoid pillowing around the active electrode. With fibrotic invasive endometriosis, blunt or sharp dissection with scissors is necessary to separate normal tissue from abnormal tissue before applying the effective surgical energy to the remaining tissue tendrils held on stretch by medial traction.

Endometriosis is a disease of predictable patterns of pelvic involvement, with or without local invasion. Because of this, only a few basic techniques are necessary for successful excision anywhere in the pelvis. These techniques include superficial excision, deep excision, resection of a uterosacral ligament and ovarian cystectomy. A skilled surgeon can build on these basic techniques to include bowel resection for endometriosis which is covered in Chapter 12.

PROCEDURE

In low lithotomy and steep Trendelenburg position, laparoscopy is performed as described in Chapter 1. Once pneumoperitoneum is established, two 5.5-mm trocars are placed in the lower quadrants lateral to the inferior epigastric vessels, the one on the right for a suction-irrigator, the one on the left for an atraumatic grasper. A 3-mm monopolar scissors is passed down the operating channel of the laparoscope and connected to an electrosurgical generator supplying 90 or more watts of pure cutting current and 50 W of coagulation current controlled by foot pedals.

Superficial resection

The abnormal peritoneum (Fig.11.1) is grasped and drawn medially, elevating it away from underlying vital structures. With a "touch cut" using pure cutting current, the active electrode creates a small hole in adjacent normal peritoneum. The graspers and scissors then bluntly undermine the abnormal peritoneum (Fig. 11.2), separating it from underlying vital structures (Fig. 11.3). With a few strokes using cutting current, the abnormal tissue is excised. This technique can also be used for diffuse peritoneal lesions (Figs 11.4–11.7).

Deep resection

Some lesions of endometriosis are invasive, and retroperitoneal fibrosis can encroach on or surround vital structures such as the ureter, pelvic vessels or nerves. The principles of resection of deep disease are similar to those of superficial resections, with two important differences: (1) retroperitoneal blunt dissection is more vigorous and demanding because of the fibrosis; (2) coagulation current is most helpful retroperitoneally.

Normal peritoneum adjacent to the invasive lesion is entered with a touch cut, then

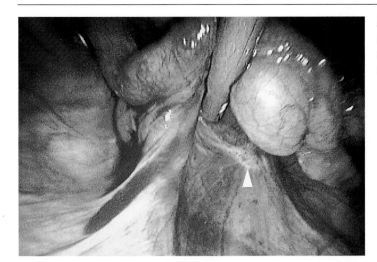

Figure 11.1 Laparoscopic view of the left adnexal region. A lesion of endometriosis (arrowhead) lies directly over the left ureter.

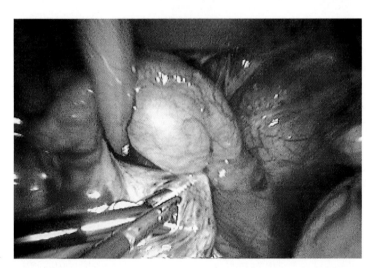

Figure 11.2 A hole has been created in normal peritoneum adjacent to the endometriotic lesion. The graspers are bluntly undermining the peritoneum, separating it from underlying vital structures.

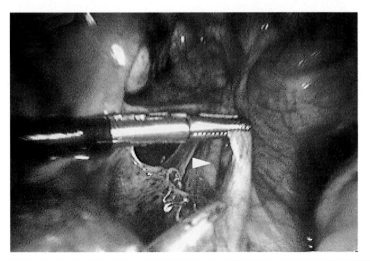

Figure 11.3 The lesion of endometriosis has been bluntly dissected away from the ureter (arrowhead) and will be excised safely with electrosurgery.

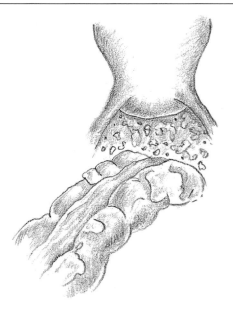

Figure 11.4 *Diffuse endometriosis of the cul de sac peritoneum. Treatment of such diffuse disease by pinpoint laser vaporization would be problematic because of the underlying rectum and the varying depths of invasion. Peritoneal resection avoids these problems.*

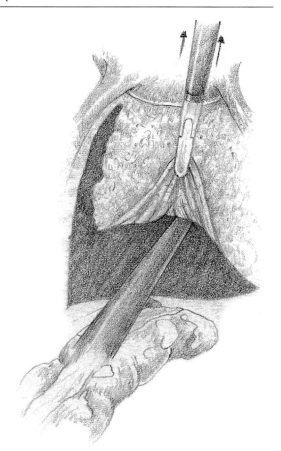

Figure 11.6 *The peritoneal incision has been extended across the cul de sac adjacent to the rectum, and traction and blunt dissection allow the peritoneum to be lifted off the underlying rectum. The longitudinal fibres of the outer muscularis are now easily seen beneath the peritoneum. The rectum is usually not readily visible beneath the peritoneum, leading to the possibility of damage with thermal ablation.*

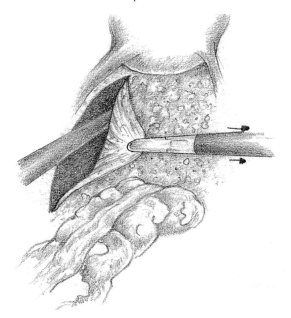

Figure 11.5 *A peritoneal incision has been made just medial to the left uterosacral ligament, and blunt dissection underneath and traction on the peritoneum allows the resection to begin.*

retroperitoneal blunt dissection is used to release normal structures from surrounding fibrosis. This will frequently require ureterolysis (Fig. 11.8) or angiolysis. The ureter is a surprisingly resilient structure which will not be injured even by vigorous blunt dissection against it. Most commonly, the invasive lesion is grasped and drawn away from the ureter, with the scissors repeatedly pushing into the space between the ureter and the invasive lesion. This will

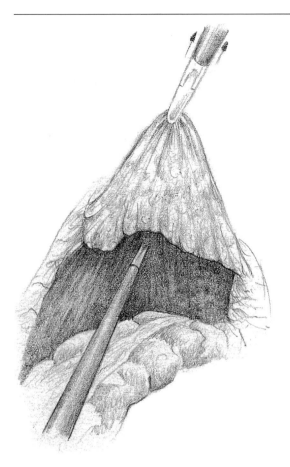

Figure 11.7 Blunt dissection is used to continue to lift the peritoneum off the rectum. When tendrils of connective tissue are visible, they can be safely severed with electrosurgery.

develop and isolate tendrils of tissue which can then be transected with short bursts of coagulation current. It is sometimes necessary to grasp the ureter firmly and pull on it to achieve counter-traction to advance the dissection. Traction can also be applied to the uterine artery but not to thin-walled veins which may tear.

In the cul de sac, invasive disease may encroach on the rectum. It is necessary to inspect the cul de sac closely in order to identify the coloration of the colon, which may blend almost imperceptibly with the coloration of normal peritoneum. Just as with ureterolysis, the abnormal tissue is forcibly separated from the rectum with blunt dissection. This can usually be applied tangentially to the bowel wall so the chance of damage to the bowel is minimal. Anteriorly, invasive disease rarely involves the bladder muscularis, so it will rarely be necessary to suture repair the bladder.

Resection of the uterosacral ligament

This technique is necessary to remove invasive disease of the uterosacral ligament and does not seem to result in defects of pelvic floor support. This technique also serves as the foundation for en bloc resection of the pelvic floor for treatment of the obliterated cul de sac in endometriosis described in Chapter 12. The key to resection of this ligament is releasing incisions made in normal peritoneum lateral and medial to the ligament using 90 W of cutting current (Fig. 11.9). These incisions allow the ureter and uterine vessels to separate from the area of the uterosacral ligament, assisted by blunt dissection laterally. A blunt probe can be used to partially undermine the ligament, particularly near its insertion into the posterior cervix. The ligament is then amputated at its insertion into the posterior cervix (Fig.11.10) and shaved off the underlying pelvic floor (Fig. 11.11) using 50 W of coagulation current. Some patients may require only isolated resection of involved peritoneum for removal of superficial disease, whereas others may require deep dissection into the sidewall for removal of all invasive disease.

Extensive resection of endometriosis may result in an increased frequency of overnight hospital stays due to nausea and vomiting, although selected patients may leave in the afternoon or evening following surgery. Medical therapy is not necessary for effective treatment of endometriosis. The first two menstrual flows may be unusually painful.

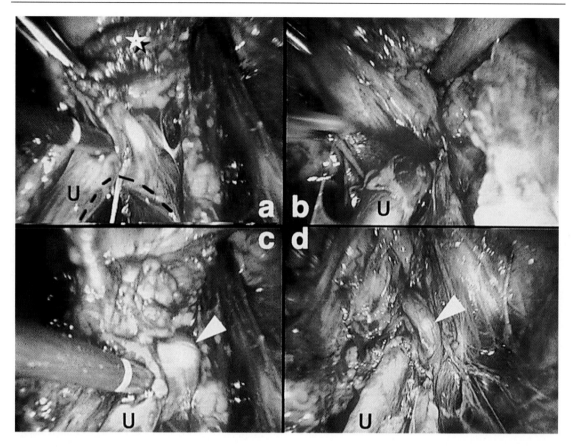

Figure 11.8 *Ureterolysis. (a) The right ureter (u) is involved with retroperitoneal fibrosis extending from a nodule of endometriosis on the right uterosacral ligament. The fibrosis is being grasped and pulled away from the ureter while the 3-mm scissors probe the plane between the ureter and the fibrosis. The path of the ureter is indicated by the dashed line. (b) The fibrotic nodule is progressively pried away from the ureter by blunt dissection, revealing tendrils of fibrotic tissue attaching the nodule to the ureter. These tendrils can be severed with a quick burst of electrosurgery. (c) Ureterolysis is carried down the ureter until the right uterine artery (arrowhead) is encountered, and it, too, must be cleared of fibrosis. (d) After complete ureterolysis, the ureter and uterine artery have been cleared of retroperitoneal fibrosis and endometriosis.*

POTENTIAL COMPLICATIONS AND THEIR PREVENTION

If electroexcision is used and the tissue to be cut is not held under strong tension, coagulation instead of cutting will occur. This not only wastes time, but may injure or obscure the underlying anatomy. Occasionally a vessel of the broad ligament may be lacerated. Since the peritoneum should invariably have been opened prior to such an injury, the ureter is frequently already exposed so that coagulation of the bleeding vessel can be accomplished safely.

CONTRAINDICATIONS

If a patient is to undergo laparoscopy, there is no known contraindication to excision other than the surgeon's inexperience. Excision can be used to treat superficial or invasive endometriosis anywhere in the body.

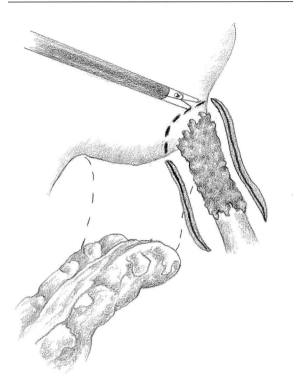

Figure 11.9 *The right uterosacral ligament has been surrounded laterally and medially by lines of peritoneal incision. The uterosacral ligament will be transected at its insertion into the posterior cervix above the invasive disease using 50 W of coagulation current* (dashed line).

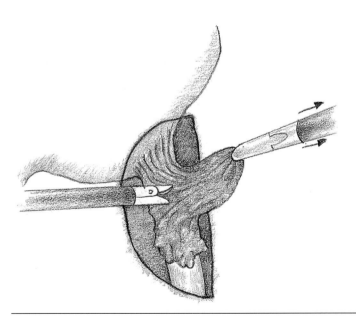

Figure 11.10 *Traction is used on the uterosacral ligament* (straight arrows) *while electrosurgery is used to shave the diseased tissue off the pelvic floor. Treatment of such invasive disease by thermal ablation would be problematic.*

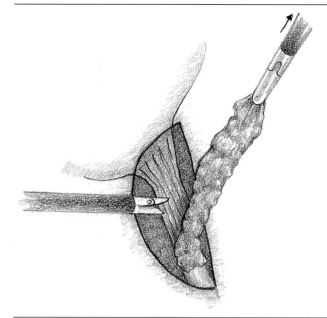

Figure 11.11 *Continued traction* (straight arrow) *allows the diseased portion of the ligament to be completely resected.*

SUGGESTED READING

Ahmed MS, Barbieri RL: Reoperation rates for recurrent ovarian endometriomas after surgical excision. *Gynecol Obstet Invest* 1997 **43**: 53–54.

Redwine DB: Conservative laparoscopic excision of endometriosis by sharp dissection: life table analysis of reoperation and persistent or recurrent disease. *Fertil Steril* 1991 **56**: 628–634.

Redwine DB: Laparoscopic excision of endometriosis by sharp dissection. In Soderstrom RA (ed). *Operative Laparoscopy, The Masters' Techniques*. Raven Press, New York, 1993, pp. 101–106.

Redwine DB: Non-laser resection of endometriosis. In Sutton CA and Diamond MP (eds) *Endoscopic Surgery for Gynaecologists*. W.B. Saunders, London, 1993, pp. 220–228.

Wood C, Maher P: Peritoneal surgery in the treatment of endometriosis – Excision or thermal ablation? *Aust NZ J Obstet Gynaecol* 1996 **36**: 190–197.

12

BOWEL RESECTION RELATED TO ENDOMETRIOSIS

David B. Redwine

Intestinal endometriosis involves the lower colon, ileum, caecum and appendix in descending order. The primary indication for bowel resection for endometriosis is to improve specific or non-specific symptoms which may be due to bowel disease. Preoperative intestinal studies carry a false negative rate of 86% since endometriosis rarely penetrates into the bowel lumen, accordingly diagnosis of bowel endometriosis is usually made surgically. If intestinal endometriosis is anticipated, a mechanical bowel prep is mandatory in case of full thickness resection. The surgeon must be familiar with the identification of all forms of endometriosis and must examine the frequently involved intestinal areas in all patients. The depth of intestinal invasion and the size and number of nodules in the intestinal area determine the type of intestinal resection to be done. The four layers of the colonic wall are serosa, outer longitudinal muscularis, inner circular muscularis, and mucosa (Fig. 12.1). The serosa is lost below the peritoneal reflection of the cul de sac. These layers can be easily separated like peeling the layers of an onion. Triple puncture laparoscopy is used by the author, and the patient is positioned with hips on the edge of the table and an intrauterine manipulator in place (Fig. 12.2).

STAGES IN THE PROCEDURE

Superficial resection

Superficial endometriosis can be grasped and the scissors cut into the serosa and outer layer of muscularis adjacent to the lesion, working from several sides so that the lesion is surrounded by a line of incision. This is advisable since otherwise the ease of dissection within the layers of the bowel wall may quickly lead the dissection past the lesion, leading to a larger than necessary defect. The defect in the bowel wall is closed with interrupted 3-0 silk suture.

Mucosal skinning

Some larger invasive lesions involve both layers of muscularis. In such cases, the scissors cut through the normal bowel wall adjacent to the nodular invasive lesion until the dissection is sufficiently deep to undermine the adjacent lesion. This initial incision is made more or less perpendicularly into the bowel wall, working with a series of small cuts rather than one large cut. Once the mucosa is encountered, the outer layers of muscularis containing the invasive lesion are dissected bluntly off the exposed mucosa. Once again, it is important to be aware of the linear extent of the lesion along the bowel wall, since it is easy to dissect far beyond. Several centimetres of mucosa can be

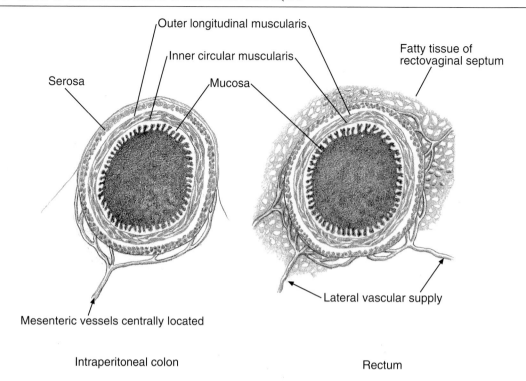

Figure 12.1 *Layers of the colonic wall. Notice that the vascular supply to the rectum lies more laterally than the blood supply to the sigmoid colon.*

exposed without entering the bowel lumen, allowing resection of large, bulky lesions. The seromuscular layers are closed with interrupted 3-0 silk sutures. Although there may be concern over inducing surgical distortion of the bowel wall by foreshortening the anterior bowel wall during suture closure, anterior muscularis defects up to 6 cm in length have been closed without producing symptoms of obstruction or obstipation.

Full thickness resection

When the submucosa is involved by fibrosis, the dissection can lead into the bowel lumen. The scissors cut into the mucosa around the nodularity, then back out through the bowel wall to the serosa. The mucosa is closed with running 3-0 chromic and the seromuscular layers are closed with interrupted 3-0 silk suture. Occasionally, a silk suture may penetrate the lumen without the surgeon's knowledge, but this is no

cause for great concern since some bowel surgeons repair full thickness bowel injuries with a single layer of through-and-through interrupted silk sutures.

Obliteration of the cul de sac

When the rectosigmoid is adherent to the posterior cervix, such obliteration of the cul de sac usually signifies the presence of invasive disease of the uterosacral ligaments, cul de sac, and frequently the anterior rectal wall (Figs 12.3 and 12.4). Therefore, simply releasing the bowel from its adherence to the posterior cervix does nothing to treat invasive endometriosis. An en bloc resection of the pelvic floor combined with partial or full-thickness bowel resection is necessary to ensure complete removal of all disease.

Releasing incisions are created in normal peritoneum lateral and parallel to the uterosacral ligaments (Figs 12.4 and 12.5).

a.

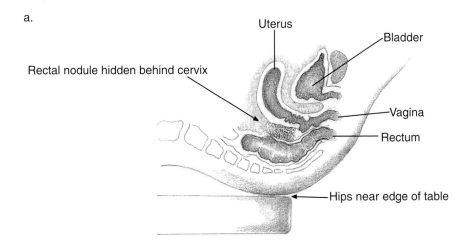

Uterus

Bladder

Rectal nodule hidden behind cervix

Vagina

Rectum

Hips near edge of table

Figure 12.2 *Patient positioning* (a) *and an intrauterine manipulator* (b) *are important for identifying and treating endometriosis.*

b.

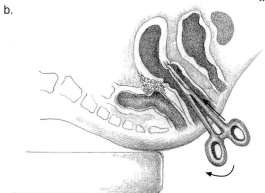

The ureter and uterine artery and vein are bluntly dissected laterally, and the peritoneal incision usually results in automatic separation of these vital structures from the uterosacral ligament. Another set of vessels courses up the posterolateral vaginal wall, ascending just lateral to the uterosacral ligaments and anastomosing with the uterine artery and vein. It is important to anticipate these vessels to avoid injury to them. A transverse incision is made across the posterior cervix above the line of adherence of the colon (Figs 12.4 and 12.6), and then an intrafascial dissection is carried down the posterior cervix toward the rectovaginal septum (Fig. 12.7). A layer of cervix approximately 2–4 mm in thickness is taken from the posterior body of the cervix in order to remove any invasive disease in this region. Occasionally the surgeon will see the release of small pockets of brownish fluid, indicating that invasive disease extends even deeper. In such cases, the dissection must proceed even deeper into the cervical stroma, although care must be taken not to enter the cervical canal. If entry into the cervical canal occurs, it must be repaired in layers to avoid a cervicoperitoneal fistula.

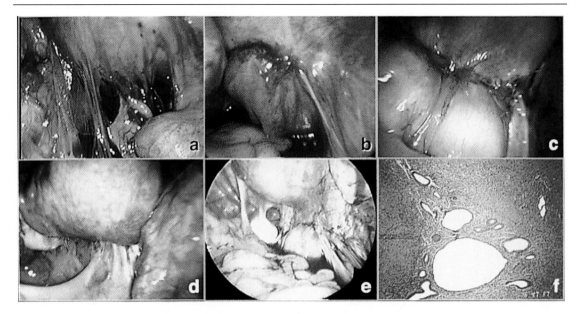

Figure 12.3 *Obliteration of the cul de sac in endometriosis.* (a) *Although the cul de sac in this patient is obscured by curtains of filmy adhesions, this is not obliteration of the cul de sac, but simply adhesions obscuring the posterior pelvis. The cul de sac in this case was actually free and normal. Adhesions like this are sometimes due to previous surgery or infection.* (b) *Complete obliteration of the cul de sac. Notice the rectum is adherent to the posterior cervix, with a round bulge in the rectal wall indicating a high likelihood of invasion of the rectal wall by endometriosis. Slight haemorrhage is present, but this represents a bloody reaction to endometriosis, not endometriosis itself.* (c) *Complete obliteration of the cul de sac, again with a round bulge to the rectal wall due to invasive colonic endometriosis.* (d) *Complete obliteration of the cul de sac. The rectum was not invaded by endometriosis in this case, and there is no round bulge of the rectal wall.* (e) *Complete obliteration of the cul de sac is occasionally accompanied by bloody peritoneal fluid.* (f) *Photomicrograph of endometriosis in the middle of an obliterated cul de sac. The surrounding fibromuscular reaction is characteristic of obliteration of the cul de sac.*

Once the fatty tissue of the rectovaginal septum has been encountered, the incisions lateral to the uterosacral ligaments are now carried around the posterior extent of invasive disease of these ligaments, then across the normal serosa of the anterior bowel wall proximal to the invasive lesion. The obliterated cul de sac remains obliterated, but it is now isolated in the centre of the pelvis attached to the anterior bowel wall (Fig. 12.8). The lateral fatty attachments of the rectosigmoid are severed, thus restoring complete mobility to the involved segment of bowel. The bulky nodular lesion (composed of the posterior cervix, uterosacral ligaments, obliterated cul de sac and anterior bowel wall) can now be removed from the bowel by superficial resection, mucosal skinning, or full thickness resection with repair as discussed above . When full thickness resection has occurred, the lesion can be removed transanally. When rectovaginal endometriosis penetrates the vaginal epithelium, the vaginal lesion is first circumscribed with a line of incision into the fatty rectovaginal septum. Then, the laparoscopic dissection down the posterior cervix will easily encounter the dissection which has been prepared from below (Fig. 12.9).

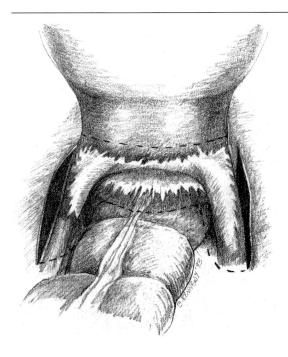

Figure 12.4 *Obliteration of the cul de sac signifies the presence of invasive endometriosis of the pelvic floor, including the anterior bowel wall in most patients.*

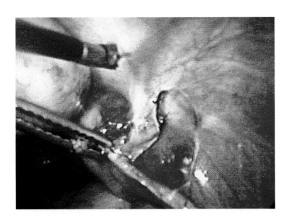

Figure 12.5 *Treatment of obliteration of the cul de sac begins by creating peritoneal incisions lateral and parallel to the uterosacral ligaments. This is the case seen in Fig. 12.3(b), with the peritoneal incision being created lateral to the right uterosacral ligament.*

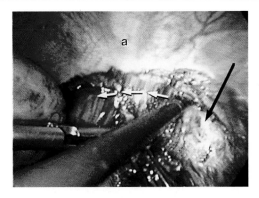

Figure 12.6. *After creation of peritoneal incisions lateral to each uterosacral ligament, a transverse incision is created across the posterior cervix (a) above the line of adherence of the bowel. An intrafascial dissection is carried down the back of the cervix toward the rectovaginal septum. In this case, the right side of the rectovaginal septum has been quickly encountered and is identified by yellow fatty tissue (black arrow).* The white arrows *indicate the line of incision which will be continued down the posterior cervix until all nodular endometriosis has been separated from the cervix. It is important not to try to find a plane of dissection between the rectum and cervix, since it is frequently indistinct and this will only leave a broad raw area with invasive endometriosis still present on the cervix, uterosacral ligaments and bowel wall.*

Segmental bowel resection

When a very large bowel nodule is present, or when several nodules are in close proximity, the defect in the anterior bowel wall resulting from local resection might be impossible to close primarily. In such rare cases, a laparoscopic segmental bowel resection with stapled anastomosis can be considered. Although this is technically feasible, its application would typically follow a potentially long and difficult pelvic dissection to remove all other pelvic disease and to free the involved bowel segment. Laparoscopic segmental bowel resection itself is a challenging procedure which may take several hours to accomplish. Most surgeons would serve their patients better by

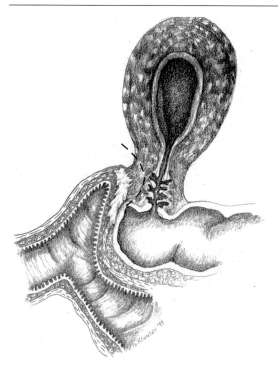

Figure 12.7 *Sagittal section drawing showing the intrafascial dissection created down the posterior cervix. This increases the likelihood of complete removal of invasive disease. No attempt should be made to separate the rectum from the outer layer of cervix, instead remove the outer layer of the cervix itself.*

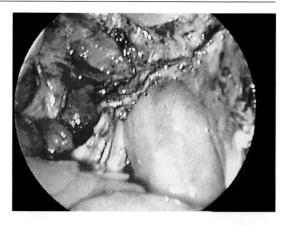

Figure 12.8 *The transverse incision across the posterior cervix has been completed and the rectovaginal septum has been partially developed. After further development of the distal rectovaginal septum, the entire nodular mass of invasive endometriosis will fall away from the cervix and lie completely isolated on the anterior rectal wall. The cul de sac remains obliterated and will be removed en bloc by rectal wall resection.*

performing all laparoscopic surgery possible then opening the abdomen with a limited incision to complete the bowel resection (laparoscopically assisted bowel resection.)

An easier technique is laparoscopically assisted transvaginal segmental resection (Fig. 12.10). The affected segment of bowel is separated laparoscopically from its mesentery using monopolar electrosurgery and delivered through the vagina to the introitus where segmental resection and sutured anastomosis are performed. Rectal and sigmoid lesions can be treated by this method. A rectal pull-through technique has been described but may be associated with an increased risk of rectal dysfunction about which patients should be warned.

Resection of the ileum

The general principles of partial thickness resection, mucosal skinning and full thickness resection discussed above also apply to the ileum. Since the ileal wall is thinner than the colonic wall, full-thickness penetration during surgery is more likely. The mucosa can be closed with a separate suture of 3-0 chromic, and the seromuscularis with interrupted 3-0 silk.

POTENTIAL COMPLICATIONS

Of 486 patients with biopsy-proven bowel endometriosis in the author's private practice, 301 have undergone laparoscopic treatment of bowel lesions, including 90 patients with full-thickness resections and 14 with segmental resections with end-to-end anastomosis. Two patients had an aborted laparoscopic segmental resection due to technical difficulty with the stapler and required a laparotomy to complete the pro-

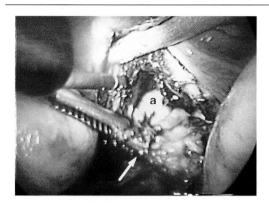

Figure 12.9 *In patients with invasion of the vagina by endometriosis, incisions are created vaginally before laparoscopy starts. These incisions are carried only into the normal fatty tissue of the rectovaginal septum adjacent to the invasive endometriosis as well as immediately adjacent to the posterior cervix, with no attempt being made to dissect the invasive disease from a vaginal approach. Laparoscopically, the transverse incision down the posterior cervix will encounter the vaginal incision adjacent to the cervix, and removal of the vaginal endometriosis will be easy due to the vaginal wall incisions already created. This view shows the normal distal vaginal epithelium* (a), *with the graspers grasping the rectovaginal nodule which was invading the posterior vaginal fornix* (arrow).

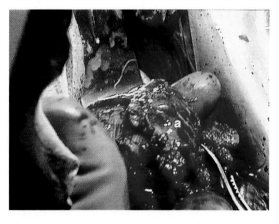

Figure 12.10 *Laparoscopically assisted transvaginal segmental bowel resection allows a minimally invasive means of treating significant intestinal endometriosis. After laparoscopic separation of the affected segment of bowel from its mesentery, the diseased loop of bowel is prolapsed through a posterior colpotomy for segmental resection and anastomosis on the perineum. Here the surgeon's fingers are behind the diseased loop of bowel and the ring forceps are on a large nodule of intestinal endometriosis*

cedure. One patient had a low-grade post-operative fever which responded to intravenous and oral antibiotics. Another, who underwent a long (7 hours) procdure, had bilateral peroneal nerve palsies which resolved after several months. A patient with a prolonged bleeding time had a small, painful pelvic haematoma which resolved after 10 days of observation.

Serious complications have been rare. One patient undergoing partial thickness resection without suture repair had late perforation of her sigmoid colon 6 days post-operatively which was repaired laparoscopically within 4 h of occurrence with no further problems. Another who had undergone a full thickness resection of the rectum had a delayed leak and required a temporary colostomy which has since been reversed. In this patient, the suture line had been proved airtight with underwater air pressure examination and watertight by injection of povidone iodine rectally. A sigmoidoscopy was then performed to try to visualize the suture line, and it is possible that this may have caused disruption of the intact suture repair. Consequently, underwater air pressure examination is sufficient to confirm intact bowel closure.

Monopolar electrosurgery on the bowel is safe in experienced hands when high current density is used, such as 90 W pure cutting current delivered through the tip of 3-mm scissors. This results in a quick, clean cut with no lateral thermal spread. Low current density is dangerous since it results in coagulation and lateral thermal spread. In more than 1300 laparoscopic procedures performed by the author using monopolar electrosurgery, the incidence of complications related to electrosurgery has been zero.

CONTRAINDICATIONS

There are no specific medical contraindications to laparoscopic bowel resection if a patient is already to undergo laparoscopy. Lack of a bowel prep is a relative contraindication, since penetration of the unprepared bowel carries an increased risk of postoperative infection. However, in skilled hands, mucosal skinning can be performed safely without a bowel prep. Inexperience of the surgeon and inability to suture laparoscopically are other potential contraindications to laparoscopic bowel surgery.

SUGGESTED READING

Redwine DB: Laparoscopic en bloc resection for treatment of the obliterated cul de sac in endometriosis. *J Reprod Med* 1992 **37**: 695–698.

Redwine DB: Laparoscopic excision of endometriosis by sharp dissection. In Soderstrom RA (ed) *Operative Laparoscopy, The Masters' Techniques.* Raven Press, New York, 1993, pp. 101–106.

Redwine DB, Sharpe DR: Laparoscopic segmental resection of the sigmoid colon for endometriosis. *J Laparoendoscopic Surg* 1991 **1**: 217–220.

Redwine DB, Koning M, Sharpe DR: Laparoscopically assisted transvaginal segmental bowel resection for endometriosis. *Fertil Steril* 1996 **65**: 193–197.

Reich H, McGlynn F, Salvat J: Laparoscopic treatment of cul-de-sac obliteration secondary to retrocervical deep fibrotic endometriosis. *J Reprod Med* 1991 **36**: 516–522.

13

LAPAROSCOPIC TREATMENT OF POLYCYSTIC OVARIAN SYNDROME

Togas Tulandi

The oldest treatment for anovulatory infertility associated with polycystic ovarian syndrome (PCOS) is bilateral ovarian wedge resection. This procedure, however is associated with a high incidence of periadnexal adhesions that may jeopardize fertility. Clomiphene citrate is today the first line of treatment for anovulation, but 25% of anovulatory women do not respond to clomiphene. Those who do not respond to clomiphene may be treated with gonadotropins or pulsatile luteinizing hormone releasing hormone, but neither modality of treatment is universally successful. An alternative surgical treatment is laparoscopic ovarian drilling. This technique is less invasive than ovarian wedge resection by laparotomy, is associated with less adhesion formation and produces excellent results. The average ovulation rate after ovarian drilling is 80% with a conception rate of 60%.

The ovary is first immobilized with a grasping forceps (Fig. 13.1). Ovarian drilling can be done using a unipolar needle electrode or laser. The use of an insulated unipolar needle electrode is associated with less adhesion formation and higher pregnancy rate than laser. As most of the uninsulated part of the needle is inside the ovary, the risk of sparking is reduced. The needle is inserted as perpendicular as possible to the ovarian surface. A short duration of cutting current of 100 W is used to aid the entry of the needle.

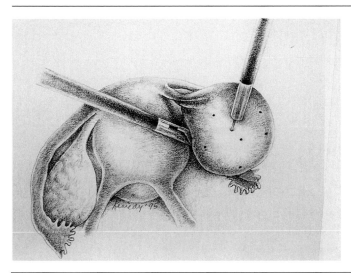

Figure 13.1 Ovarian drilling using an insulated unipolar needle electrode. *From Tulandi T: Operative laparoscopy, In Thompson JD and Rock JA (eds) Te Linde's Update in Operative Gynecology, 1997. Reproduced with permission.*

Figure 13.2a

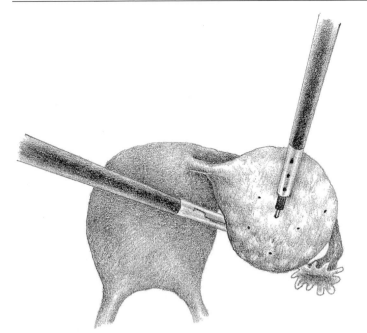

Figure 13.2b

Figure 13.2 *Ovarian drilling of the anterior aspect of the ovary.*

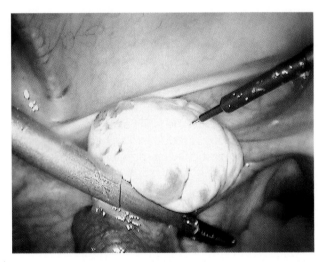

The whole length of the needle (8 mm) is inserted into the ovary and it is activated with 40 W of coagulating current for 2 seconds at each point. The anterior surface is exposed by "flipping" the ovary upward with a forceps (Fig. 13.2). Depending on the size of the ovary, 10–15 punctures per ovary are created (Fig. 13.3). Liberal irrigation of the pelvic cavity to remove necrotic debris and carbon materials should be done at the completion of ovarian drilling.

COMPLICATIONS AND THEIR PREVENTION

Excessive drilling may cause ovarian atrophy and premature menopause. Creating more than 20 craters per ovary and drilling the ovarian hilum should be avoided. This may jeopardize the blood supply to the ovary and may also cause bleeding. Damage to the ovarian surface can cause periovarian adhesion that may further decrease

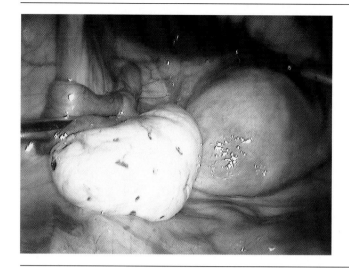

Figure 13.3 *Appearance of the ovary after ovarian drilling*

fertility. Accordingly, the needle electrode should be inserted perpendicular to the ovarian surface until its insulated part is inside the ovary. This procedure should be limited to women who are resistant to clomiphene who for some reason cannot be treated with gonadotropin or luteinizing hormone releasing hormone.

SUGGESTED READING

Donesky BW, Adashi EY: Surgically induced ovulation in the polycystic ovary syndrome: wedge resection revisited in the age of laparoscopy. *Fertil Steril* 1995 **63**: 439.

Farhi J, Soules S, Jacobs HS: Effect of laparoscopic ovarian electrocautery on ovarian response and outcome of treatment with gonadotropins in clomiphene citrate-resistant patients with polycystic ovary syndrome. *Fertil Steril* 1995 **64**: 930–935.

Gjönnaes H: Ovarian electrocautery in the treatment of women with polycystic ovary syndrome (PCOS). Factors affecting the results. *Acta Obstet Gynecol Scand* 1994 **73**: 407.

Naether OGJ, Fischer R, Weise HC, Geiger-Kötzler L, Delfs T, Rudolf K: Laparoscopic electrocoagulation of the ovarian surface in infertile patients with polycystic ovarian disease. *Fertil Steril* 1993 **60**: 88–94.

Tulandi T, Watkin K, Tan SL: Reproductive performance and three dimensional ultrasound volume determination of polycystic ovaries following laparoscopic ovarian drilling. *Int J Fertil* 1997 **42**: 436–440.

14

LAPAROSCOPIC PRESACRAL NEURECTOMY

David B. Redwine

Presacral neurectomy (PSN) has been performed since 1899 in order to relieve midline pelvic pain or severe uterine cramping with menses. Despite the use of the term "presacral", most of the procedure is actually done on the ventral aspect of the body of the fifth lumbar vertebra as well as in the superior hollow of the sacrum. The simple laparoscopic technique developed by the author is presented below.

STAGES IN THE PROCEDURE

A triple puncture technique is used, with a 10-mm operating laparoscope inserted through the umbilicus, a 5-mm grasper inserted in a left lower quadrant port lateral to the inferior epigastric vessels, and a suction irrigator inserted through a right lower quadrant port. A 3-mm monopolar scissors is passed down the channel of the operating laparoscope. Laparoscopic PSN should precede pelvic surgery because the presacral tissue can become oedematous and the important landmarks obscured if lengthy pelvic surgery occurs before the PSN. The patient is placed in steep Trendelenburg position and the small bowel placed in the upper abdomen. The operating table is rolled to the left, displacing the sigmoid laterally. The suction irrigator is used to push the sigmoid even further laterally.

The left common iliac vein and bifurcation of the vena cava extend a variable distance caudad to the aortic bifurcation (Fig. 14.1) and can be identified by eliciting the waterbed sign. Light percussion with a blunt probe of the peritoneum over the left common iliac vein will cause the low pressure blood in the vein to bounce like a waterbed. The left common iliac vein frequently lies nearly in the midline of the promontory of the fifth lumbar vertebra, obscured by the overlying peritoneum and presacral tissue, and represents the major vascular structure which is most likely to be injured during the performance of a PSN. The right common iliac vein lies beneath the right common iliac artery, so injury is less likely.

The peritoneum is grasped in the midline and elevated away from the underlying vital structures (Fig. 14.2). A touch cut is created in the peritoneum with the 3-mm scissors using 90 W of pure cutting current. The incision is extended transversely (Fig. 14.3) to the right common iliac vessels near the ureteral crossing, and to the edge of the sigmoid mesentery on the left. The left ureter will rarely be seen during the procedure since it is hidden lateral to the vessels of the sigmoid mesentery. Electrosurgical cutting is performed with the closed tip of the scissors, or with the edge of one blade. The scissors are not operated in a mechanical fashion since this will result in excessive coagulation effect rather than a clean cut.

After the transverse peritoneal incision is

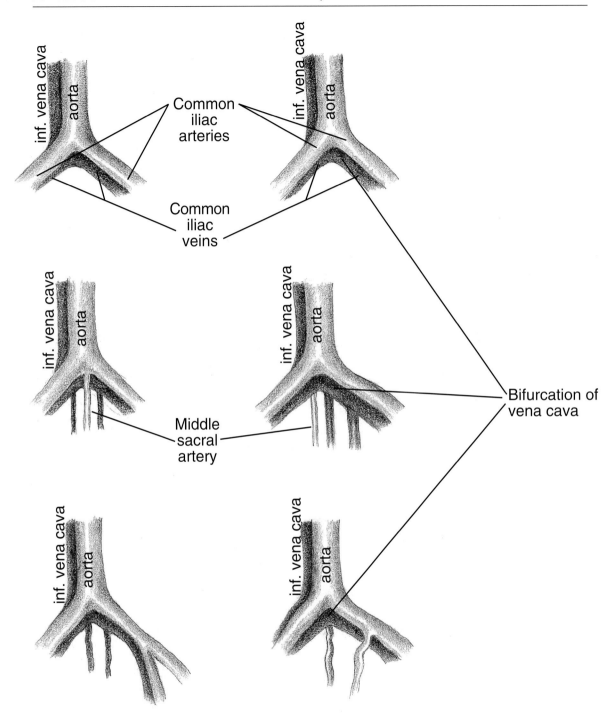

Figure 14.1 *The vascular anatomy of the presacral space can be highly variable. Not all patients have identifiable presacral vessels, whereas others may have multiple, large presacral veins.*

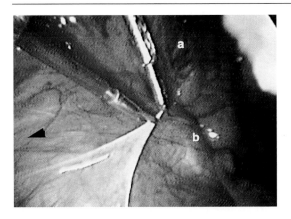

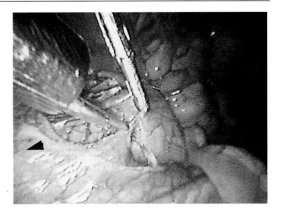

Figure 14.2 *The peritoneum over the dorsal body of L5 is grasped and elevated away from the underlying vital structures. A pair of 3-mm monopolar scissors is used with 90 W of pure cutting current to create a transverse peritoneal incision. The black arrowhead in each figure lies in the midline and indicates the direction toward the head of the patient.*

Figure 14.4 *The presacral tissue is grasped and elevated, then transected with 50 W of coagulation current passed down the 3-mm monopolar scissors. The tissue is cut by touching the tip of the scissors to the tissue.*

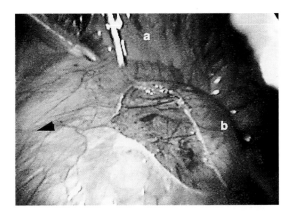

Figure 14.3 *The transverse peritoneal incision has been created from the edge of the sigmoid mesentery on the left to the right common iliac vessels.*

made a superficial layer of presacral tissue is grasped and elevated up and away from the underlying vascular structures (Fig. 14.4), allowing the surgeon to confirm visually that no vascular structures are being elevated. The 3-mm scissors using 50 W of coagulation current are used to transect only the elevated tissue, working near the

rostral edge of the peritoneal incision. Working from left to right in successively deeper layers, the presacral tissue is grasped, elevated and touch cut. By transecting the presacral tissue in multiple small bites, damage to underlying vascular structures can be avoided. Since it is sometimes impossible to distinguish neural tissue from fat or lymphatic tissue, it is necessary to transect all presacral tissue from the base of the sigmoid mesentery on the left to the right common iliac vessels and ureter on the right. Presacral veins can sometimes be found feeding into the left common iliac vein or into the bifurcation of the vena cava (Fig. 14.5). These veins can be spared by gently dissecting the tissue off them. Not all patients have identifiable presacral veins, and a middle sacral artery is even less commonly found (Fig. 14.1).

Once the presacral tissue has been transected, its caudal cut edge can be grasped and elevated, and the presacral tissue dissected away from the periosteum and presacral vessels for several centimetres down the hollow of the sacrum. The presacral tissue is then bluntly stripped from the overlying peritoneum (Fig. 14.6) and transected distally using 50 W of coagulation current.

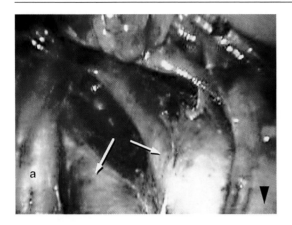

Figure 14.5 *The vascular anatomy of the presacral space is variable. The edge of the sigmoid mesentery (a) is seen on the left. Some patients may have multiple large presacral veins (arrows).*

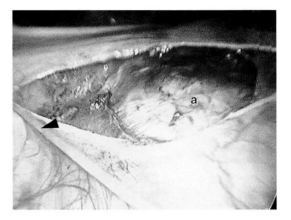

Figure 14.7 *The presacral neurectomy has been completed. The bare periosteum of L5 is seen (a), with the edge of the bifurcation of the vena cava seen next to the cut edge of peritoneum to the left. Notice the complete absence of presacral vessels in this patient.*

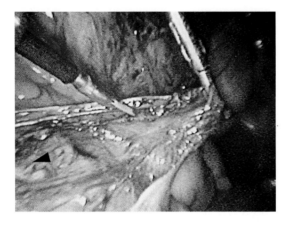

Figure 14.6 *After the presacral tissue has been transected down to the presacral vessels or to the periosteum, the presacral tissue is dissected bluntly inferiorly as shown here. It will then be stripped from the overlying peritoneum and transected distally to obtain a specimen. Notice the small venous and arterial structures on the periosteum.*

At this point of the procedure, care must be taken not to coagulate blindly through the overlying peritoneum since the sigmoid colon is always present immediately behind the peritoneum. At the conclusion of the procedure, the periosteum and any presacral vessels have been laid bare from the base of the sigmoid mesentery to the right common iliac vessels (Fig. 14.7).

COMPLICATIONS AND THEIR PREVENTION

Damage to the left common iliac vein or presacral veins is likely to occur if the presacral tissue is transected with imprecise energy sources such as the argon beam coagulator or carbon dioxide laser. If these energy sources are used, a backstop is recommended to protect the major vessels. If inadequate retroperitoneal dissection has been performed, or if large bundles of presacral tissue are grasped greedily, damage to surrounding structures is more likely to occur. Vigorous dissection in the sigmoid mesentery can result in significant bleeding, and subsequent coagulation to control bleeding could damage the hidden left ureter.

Postoperatively, patients may rarely mention a decreased sense of bladder fullness related to interruption of sympathetic

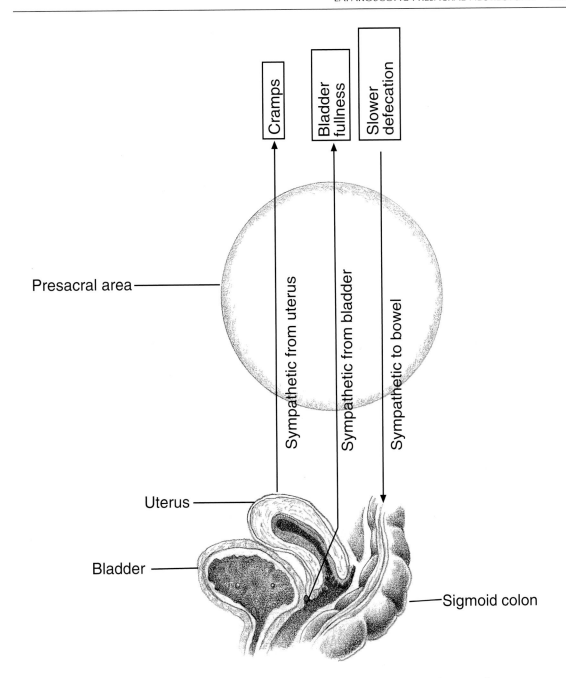

Figure 14.8 *Sympathetic nerves that are severed by a presacral neurectomy. Some patients may report a decreased sensation of bladder fullness, whereas others may notice a decrease in constipation.*

nerves from the bladder. Sympathetics to the sigmoid are severed during PSN, so some patients may be less constipated following surgery (Fig. 14.8). Despite occasional reports in the literature, constipation is not anatomically predictable following a PSN. Urinary urgency is rarely seen. The majority of patients have no change in bowel or bladder function.

CONTRAINDICATIONS

Although there are no specific contraindications, obese patients have more retroperitoneal fatty tissue in the presacral area. This can increase the difficulty of surgery and rarely may cause abandonment of the procedure.

SUGGESTED READING

Jaboulay M: Le traitement de la nevralgie pelvienne par la paralysie du sympathique sacre. *Lyon Med* 1899 **90**: 102–108.

Malinak LR: Operative management of pelvic pain. *Clin Obstet Gynecol* 1980 **23**: 191–200.

Perez JJ: Laparoscopic presacral neurectomy. Results of the first 25 cases. *J Reprod Med* 1990 **35**: 625–630.

Redwine DB, Perez JJ: Laparoscopic presacral neurectomy. In Soderstrom RA (ed) *Operative Laparoscopy, The Masters' Techniques*. Raven Press, New York, 1993 pp. 157–60.

Tjaden B, Schlaff WD, Kimball A, Rock JA: The efficacy of presacral neurectomy for the relief of midline dysmenorrhea. *Obstet Gynecol* 1990 **76**: 89–91.

15

LAPAROSCOPIC UTERINE NERVE ABLATION (LUNA)

Togas Tulandi

The sensory nerve fibres from the uterus and cervix traverse the Frankenhauser plexus which is located in, under and around the attachment of uterosacral ligaments to the posterior wall of the cervix. The pain stimuli are conducted to the sacral sympathetic plexus by way of nerve roots S-2,3 and 4. Ablation of the uterosacral ligaments disrupts the continuity of these nerve fibres. Although, pain relief has been reported in about 70% of patients treated, the efficacy of this procedure is questionable. Currently, LUNA is rarely performed in our institution.

PROCEDURE

Because the ureter is located close to the uterosacral ligament, the posterior broad ligaments should be carefully inspected to identify the course of the ureters. They are usually located 1–2 cm lateral to the uterosacral ligaments. Peristaltic movements of the ureters can be elicited by touching the ureters with atraumatic forceps. The uterosacral ligaments are exposed by elevating the uterus with a uterine manipulator. Sometimes, the ligaments are attenuated and not clearly defined. In this situation, either a suction irrigator or laparoscopic forceps are pushed against the mid-posterior aspect of the cervix to tent up the ligaments (Fig. 15.1).

The course of the ureters is inspected again and transection of the uterosacral ligaments is done using laser (power density $10\,000\,W/cm^2$) or unipolar cautery scissors. Transection is done perpendicular to the ligaments as close to the cervix as possible at their attachment to the cervix. A crater 0.5 cm deep is created. Attention should be given not to injure the ureters, blood vessels on the lateral aspect of the ligaments and the rectum. Interruption of crossing nerve fibres between the two ligaments can be done by lasering or electrocoagulating the area between the two craters superficially. At the completion of the procedure, the pelvic cavity is irrigated to remove the necrotic debris and the carbon material produced. "Examination under water" is performed to ascertain that there is no bleeding.

POTENTIAL COMPLICATIONS AND THEIR PREVENTION

Laparoscopic uterine nerve ablation is a simple procedure, but it can lead to a catastrophic complication of transecting the ureters, rectal injury, major bleeding and even death. Ureteral injury should be immediately recognized and repaired. It is of paramount importance to identify the ureters and blood vessels lateral to the uterosacral ligaments before performing

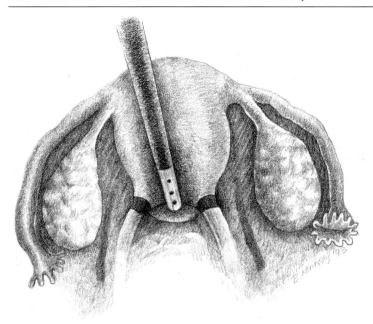

Figure 15.1 *Exposing the uterosacral ligaments with a suction irrigator during the ablation. Note the course of the ureters (dark shadow) lateral to the ligaments.*

LUNA. Bleeding can also occur because the transection is done too deep. This can usually be controlled with bipolar electro-coagulation.

SUGGESTED READING

Daniell JF: Fiberoptic laser laparoscopy. In Sutton C (ed) *Bailliere's Clinical Obstetrics and Gynaecology. Laparoscopic Surgery* 1993 **3**: 545–562.

16

LAPAROSCOPIC MYOMECTOMY

Togas Tulandi

Myoma is found in 25% of women over the age of 35. Its high prevalence suggests that not all women who harbour myoma should undergo surgery for its removal. However, those with excessive uterine bleeding, with pressure symptoms due to large uterine mass and some infertile women whose myoma is distorting the uterine cavity may require myomectomy.

LAPAROSCOPIC MYOMECTOMY

Laparoscopic excision of the myoma is done as that by laparotomy. Pedunculated myoma is removed by coagulating its pedicle with bipolar forceps or by applying two pretied ligatures (Endoloops, Rx Ethicon Inc., Sommerville, NJ; PercLoop, Laparomed, Irvine, CA) on the base of the myoma. The pedicle is cut with scissors. For intramural myoma, a solution of vasopressin (0.2 units/ml of physiological saline) is first injected into the myometrium adjacent to the myoma using a laparoscopic injection needle (Fig. 16.1). The needle is inserted into the uterine wall with the bevel facing upward. Before injecting, the anaesthetist should be notified. Although rare, its use has been associated with cardiac arrythmia and pulmonary oedema. The myometrium over the myoma is incised until the characteristic white appearance of the myoma is seen (Fig. 16.2). It is crucial to obtain a proper cleavage plane, as this will facilitate

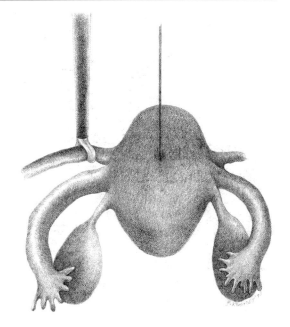

Figure 16.1 *Injection of dilute solution of vasopressin into the uterine wall overlying a myoma.*

the process of enucleation and is associated with less bleeding. Enucleation is done using laparoscopic scissors and blunt or hydrodissection. It can be aided by the use of a myoma screw that is inserted into the centre of the myoma. Blood vessels encountered during the dissection should be coagulated. The myoma is removed using a 20 mm serrated-edged macromorcellator (Fig. 16.3). The uterine incision is closed in two layers. The deeper myometrial layer is

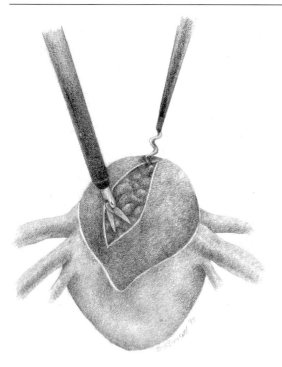

Figure 16.2 *Incision of the uterine wall.*

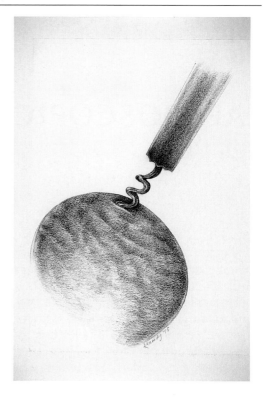

Figure 16.3 *Morcellation of a myoma with a morcellator. From Tulandi T: Operative laparoscopy. In Thompson JD and Rock JA (eds) Te Linde's Update in Operative Gynecology 1997. Reproduced with permission.*

closed using a curve needle with 0 polyglactin. The serosal layer is approximated using a ski needle with 4-0 polyglactin (Vicryl) or polydioxanone (PDS) (Fig. 16.4). The knots are tied extracorporeally or intracorporeally. Contrary to polyglactin, polydioxanone is a monofilament and is easier to handle. In the presence of a large uterine defect, approximation of the uterine incisions can be difficult. Here, a slip-knot application is helpful. The knot is made extracorporeally (Fig. 16.5) and is inserted into the abdominal cavity using a knot pusher. Once the slip knot is applied to the myometrium, the suture is cut approximately 5 cm from the tissue and another knot intracorporeally is added for reinforcement (Fig. 16.6).

Laparoscopic suturing of the uterine incisions can be time consuming. In general, laparoscopic approach should be reserved for women with pedunculated myoma, with intramural myoma of <10 cm or for those who have completed their family. Depending on the surgeon's expertise in laparoscopic suturing, laparoscopic myomectomy may result in inadequate multilayered uterine closure. Indentations of the previous myomectomy incision and uterine fistula have been noted. This might represent a structural defect. Alternatively, a laparoscopically assisted myomectomy can be done.

LAPAROSCOPICALLY ASSISTED MYOMECTOMY

Laparoscopically assisted myomectomy is done by enucleating the myoma partially by laparoscopy. The partially enucleated myoma is grasped with a claw forceps or held with a laparoscopic myoma screw that is inserted suprapubicly via a 10-mm trocar. The abdominal incision is enlarged

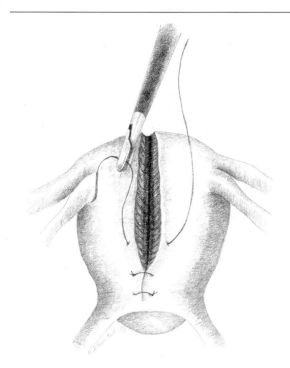

Figure 16.4 Suturing the upper layer of the myometrium.

transversely enough to accommodate the myoma and the myoma is delivered from the abdominal cavity (Figs 16.7 and 16.8). The enucleation is continued extracorporeally and the uterine defect is repaired. Closure of the uterine defect is done in two layers. The uterus is replaced into the abdominal cavity and the abdominal incision is closed. Laparoscopy is resumed and liberal irrigation of the abdominal cavity with a solution of Ringer's lactate is performed. Often, omentum is already adherent to the abdominal incision. It can be liberated with gentle traction. At the completion of the procedure, 500–1000 ml of Ringer's lactate solution is instilled into the peritoneal cavity.

The main advantage of laparoscopically assisted myomectomy is that multilayered uterine closure can be done easily without prolonging the duration of surgery. This is especially important for women with diffuse and multiple myomas. In our institution, this procedure is done when there are more than three myomas of >5 cm. Laparo-

scopically assisted myomectomy is as effective as myomectomy by laparotomy, but it is associated with a smaller incision, shorter duration of hospitalization, faster recovery and possibly less bleeding. Perhaps, this is due to the "tourniquet effect" of the abdominal wall. Because abdominal packing is not used, the return of intestinal function is faster.

Another laparoscopic approach to myoma is laparoscopic myoma coagulation (myolysis). Reduction of the size of a myoma can be done by coagulating the myoma with Nd-YAG laser or with long bipolar needle electrodes. It appears that the procedure is effective and regrowth of the myoma does not occur. Because of adhesion formation, this procedure should be reserved for women who have completed their family. Uterine rupture after this procedure has been reported.

POTENTIAL COMPLICATIONS AND THEIR PREVENTION

1. Bleeding, haematoma, breakdown of the uterine closure a few weeks after a laparoscopic myomectomy and uterine dehiscence in late pregnancy can occur. Proper multilayered closure of the uterine defect is mandatory.

2. Postmyomectomy adhesion frequently occurs. Accordingly, it is important to have good approximation of the uterine defect, to use non-reactive suture material and liberal irrigation of the abdominal cavity. Covering the uterine incision with expanded polytetrafluoroethylene (ePTFE, Preclude, GoreTex-Surgical Membrane, W.B. Gore and Associates, Inc., Flagstaff, AZ) decreases adhesion formation. Because haemostasis from the uterine incision is rarely absolute, the use of ePTFE is preferable to oxidized regenerated cellulose (ORT, TC7, Interceed, Johnson & Johnson Medical Inc., New Brunswick, NJ). Contrary to ORT, ePTFE has to be anchored to the uterus with sutures. Alternatively, a

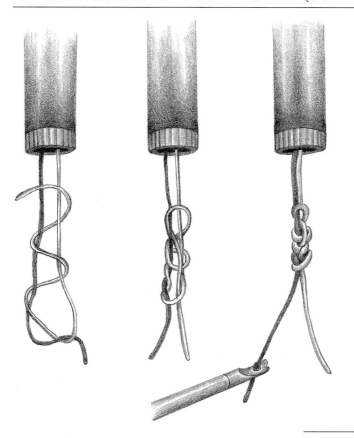

Figure 16.5 *Formation of a slip-knot. The knot is then applied to the tissue and tightened using a knot-pusher.*

second-look laparoscopy and lysis of adhesions can be done within 6 weeks after the myomectomy. The availability of small diameter laparoscopes ("mini-laparoscope") increases the feasibility of a second-look laparoscopy.

CONTRAINDICATIONS

Women with diffuse and multiple myomas, with a large leiomyomatous uterus (>18 weeks size after luteinizing hormone releasing hormone analogue (LHRHa) treatment), with a myoma larger than 10 cm and those who desire a hysterectomy are not candidates for laparoscopic myomectomy. Because of the risks of uterine rupture, myomectomy by laparotomy or laparoscopically assisted myomectomy is a better approach for surgeons who are not familiar with laparoscopic suturing.

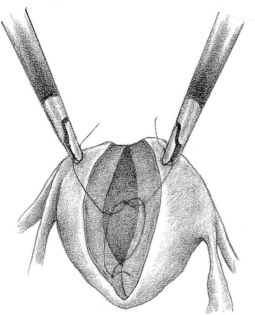

Figure 16.6 *Additional knot is supplemented for reinforcement.*

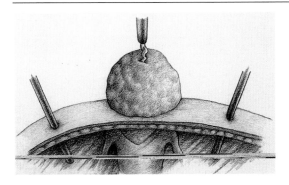

Figure 16.7

Figures 16.7 and 16.8 *Laparoscopically assisted myomectomy. A partially enucleated myoma has been delivered outside the abdominal cavity.*

SUGGESTED READING

Dubuisson JB, Cavett X, Chapron C et al.: Uterine rupture during pregnancy after laparoscopic myomectomy. *Hum Reprod* 1995 **10**: 1475–1477.

Nezhat C, Nezhat F, Bess O et al.: Laparoscopically assisted myomectomy: a report of a new technique in 57 cases. *Int J Fertil* 1994 **39**: 39–44.

Tulandi T, Laberge PY: Laparoscopic myomectomy (CD-ROM). *Human Reprod Update* 1997 **3**(4).

Tulandi T, Youssef H: Laparoscopy assisted myomectomy of large uterine myomas. *Gynaecol Endosc* 1997 **6**: 105–108.

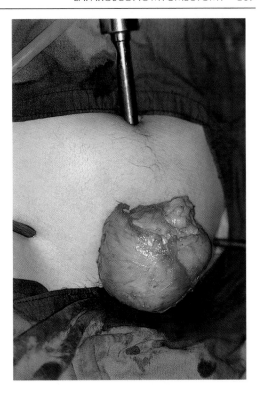

Figure 16.8

17

LAPAROSCOPIC HYSTERECTOMY

Liselotte Mettler and Kurt Semm

Laparoscopic assisted vaginal hysterectomy (LAVH) was initiated by Semm in 1982. The procedure was performed in women who had undergone many laparotomies, those who had severe intra-abdominal adhesions and in women with large benign ovarian cyst. The laparoscopic part was done to separate the adnexa from the pelvic wall and to dissect the mesosalpinx down to the cardinal ligaments. The dissection of the uterine vessels was done vaginally. In 1990, Reich reported LAVH with laparoscopic dissection of the ureters and uterine vessels and in 1991, Semm introduced classic intrafascial SEMM (serrated edged macro morcellated) hysterectomy (CISH) without colpotomy.

Laparoscopic hysterectomy and LAVH have many advantages compared to abdominal or conventional vaginal hysterectomy. Blood loss is less, hospitalization time is shorter, the incidence of ileus is less and the risk of intra-abdominal adhesions formation is reduced. Furthermore, the pelvis can be thoroughly evaluated before uterine removal and adhesions, endometriosis or leiomyoma can be removed before carrying out hysterectomy. This chapter describes several techniques of laparoscopic hysterectomy.

CLASSIC INTRAFASCIAL SUPRACERVICAL HYSTERECTOMY (CISH)

CISH can be done by laparoscopy, laparotomy or vaginally. The advantages of CISH are partial preservation of the integrity of the pelvic floor (no posterior colpotomy), preservation of blood supply to the pelvic floor, no interference with the sexual life and possible protection against cervical cancer by coring out the transformation zone.

A modification of CISH is total uterine mucosa ablation (TUMA) where the residual uterine muscle remains *in situ*. This represents an alternative method to endometrial ablation. In CISH, there are two vaginal and two laparoscopic steps.

1. *First vaginal step*: The cervix is grasped with two tenaculae that are placed at the 3 and 9 o'clock positions. Ten ml of 0.05% solution of vasopressin derivative (Rx POR-8, Ornipressin, Sandoz) is injected into the cervix. The cervix–uterine length is measured and the cervix is dilated up to bougie Hegar no. 6. A calibrated uterine resection tool (CURT) to manipulate the uterus is introduced up to the uterine fundus (Figs 17.1a and 17.2). The tenaculae are attached to the guide rod by fixation screws.

2. *First laparoscopy step* (Fig. 17.1b–e): Adnexal dissection is done by applying sutures, suture ligatures or staples until

Figure 17.1

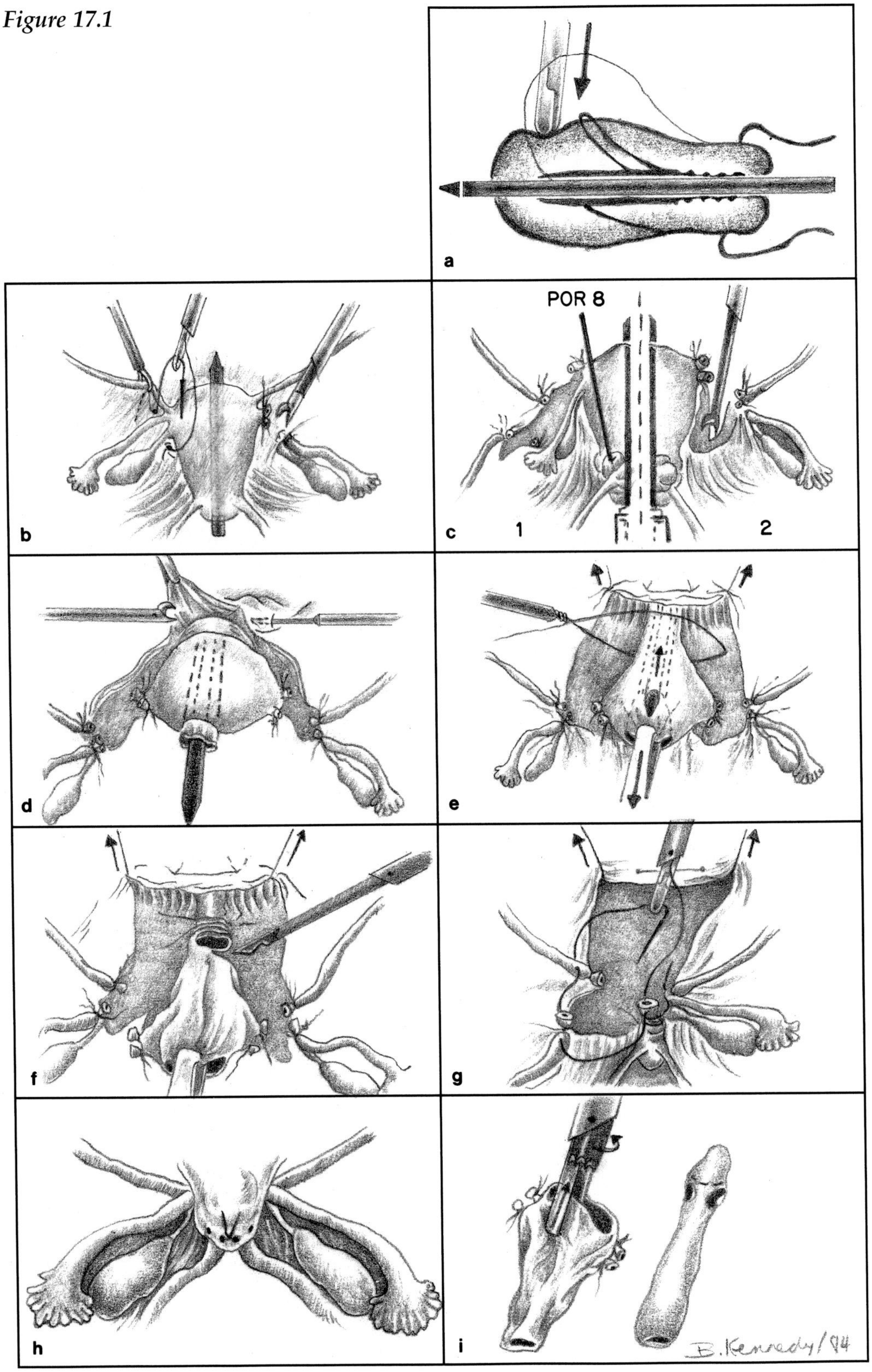

the level of the cardinal ligaments. After injection of POR-8 into the cervix, the bladder fold is dissected off the cervix with hook scissors and with a laparoscopic swab. A Roeder-loop is placed around the cervix and kept loose. The uterine vessels and ureters are not touched.

3. *Second vaginal step:* The CURT guide rod is pushed through the uterine fundus under laparoscopic control (Fig. 17.2). The inner layers of the cervix and uterus are carefully resected with the CURT by coring. The size of CURT is selected according to the measurement of the cervical diameter by ultrasound (10, 15, 20 or 24 mm). Coring is performed using a small battery device that automatically drives the coring device forward. A soon as the uterine fundus is perforated (Fig. 17.1e), the guide rod and the coring device are withdrawn and the Roeder-loop is tightened. This is to avoid loss of pneumoperitoneum. The resected uterine cylinder (Fig. 17.3) is sent for histopathological examination. The remaining cervical shell is endocoagulated with a haemostaser probe heated by an Erystop (Fig. 17.4). This is an endocoagulator with a coagulation power of 150 W and a local heat production of 120°C. The tenaculae are released and the vaginal part is completed.

4. *Second laparoscopic step* (Fig. 17.1f–i): The tightened Roeder-loop is secured with a security knot and two more loops are placed, tightened and secured. The uterine corpus is grasped with a claw forceps and is severed from the cervix with hook scissors. The cervical stump is disinfected with a disinfecting swab and endocoagulated (Fig. 17.5). The cervical stump is then suspended to the round ligaments and the visceral peritoneum is closed over the cervix. The uterus is morcellated with serrated edged macro-morcellator (SEMM) and removed from the abdominal cavity. A drain tube is inserted via a 5-mm trocar and removed after 24 h.

INTRAFASCIAL VAGINAL HYSTERECTOMY (IVH)

This is a modification of CISH where after punching out the cervical tissue, vaginal supracervical hysterectomy is performed in the usual manner. Here, the uterosacral ligaments remain and only an anterior colpotomy is performed.

LAPAROSCOPY-ASSISTED VAGINAL HYSTERECTOMY (LAVH) AND TOTAL LAPAROSCOPY-ASSISTED VAGINAL HYSTERECTOMY (TLAVH)

One of the primary purposes of LAVH is to convert an abdominal hysterectomy to a

---

Figure 17. 1 (opposite) *Steps for CISH:*

a. *Transcervical–transuterine perforation of the uterine fundus with the guide rod of the calibrated uterine resection tool (CURT).*

b. *Adnexal separation from the uterus after securing with suture–ligatures and extracorporeal knot tying.*

c. *Infiltration of the cervix and the bladder fold with the vasopressin derivative POR-8 and further dissection of the broad ligament.*

d. *Aquadissection and dissection of the bladder fold.*

e. *Placement of a Roeder-loop around the cervix and coring the transcervical–transuterine cylinder with the CURT.*

f. *Supracervical separation of the uterus with scissors.*

g. *Suspension of the cervical stump to the round ligaments bilaterally.*

h. *Peritoneal closure with a continuous suture.*

i. *Uterine morcellation with the serrated edged macro-morcellator (SEMM).*

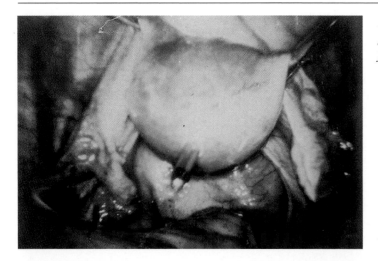

Figure 17.2 Placement of CURT guide rod through the uterine fundus.

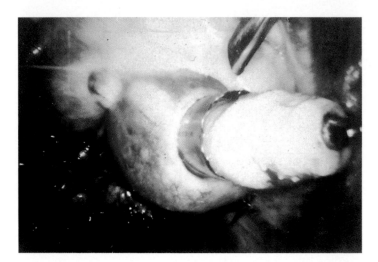

Figure 17.3 Laparoscopic view of resection of the cervico-uterine mucosa.

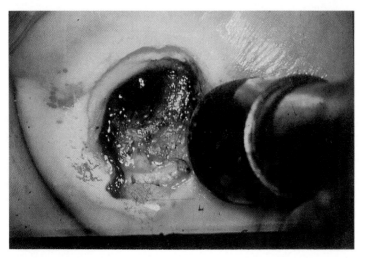

Figure 17.4 Endocoagulation of the remaining part of the cervix with Erystop.

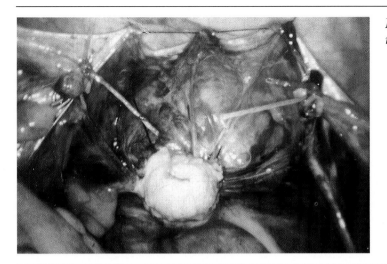

Figure 17.5 *Cervical stump after resection of the uterine corpus.*

vaginal procedure. Thus, essentially any condition that prevents a vaginal hysterectomy, but can be solved laparoscopically, represents an indication for LAVH. LAVH can be done with anterior or posterior colpotomy incision. The difference between LAVH and TLAVH is in the extent of laparoscopic dissection. In LAVH, the laparoscopic dissection along the cervix is stopped some distance above the uterine vessels. In TLAVH, dissection of the uterine vessels and the uterus is done laparoscopically and the vaginal part is only to remove the uterus.

Laparosopically assisted vaginal hysterectomy (LAVH)

LAVH with anterior colpotomy is also called laparoscopic Doderlein hysterectomy (Fig. 17.6). Haemostasis is done either with electrocautery, sutures, clips or staples. The optic trocar is inserted through the umbilicus and additional trocars further down. The patient is placed in a deep Trendelenburg position with shoulder braces.

The course of the ureter should always be followed before and throughout the procedure. If the ovaries are to be removed, an EndoGauge measuring instrument is placed on the infundibulopelvic ligament to determine the proper Multifire Endo GIA-30 cartridge for transecting the ligament. We usually place the Vascular Endo GIA stapler via the left lower quadrant port to transect the right infundibulopelvic ligament. A second stapler is placed via the ipsilateral port to transect the broad and the round ligaments. If the ovaries are to be retained, transection is done on the utero-ovarian ligaments. First the camera is moved to the right lower quadrant port and the stapler is inserted through the 12-mm umbilical port. A second stapler is placed parallel to the uterine fundus incorporating the round ligament and the upper portion of the broad ligament.

The bladder flap is developed using sharp dissection with scissors. This can be facilitated by hydrodissection using solution of 0.05% POR-8. The bladder is dissected off the lower uterine segment and the cervix until the endopelvic fascia overlying the cervix is identified. This frequently requires the use of an endoscopic swab (a "peanut" gauze). Haemostasis especially in the area of the bladder pillar should be secured. The course of the ureters is again followed. The last application of the stapler is on each side of the uterus parallel to the cervix stopping approximately 3 mm above the uterine artery. Note that the Multifire Endo GIA-30 spans 8 mm from the inside of the cartridge to the outside row of staples and often the space between the cervix and the ureter is less than 8 mm. Therefore, application of the

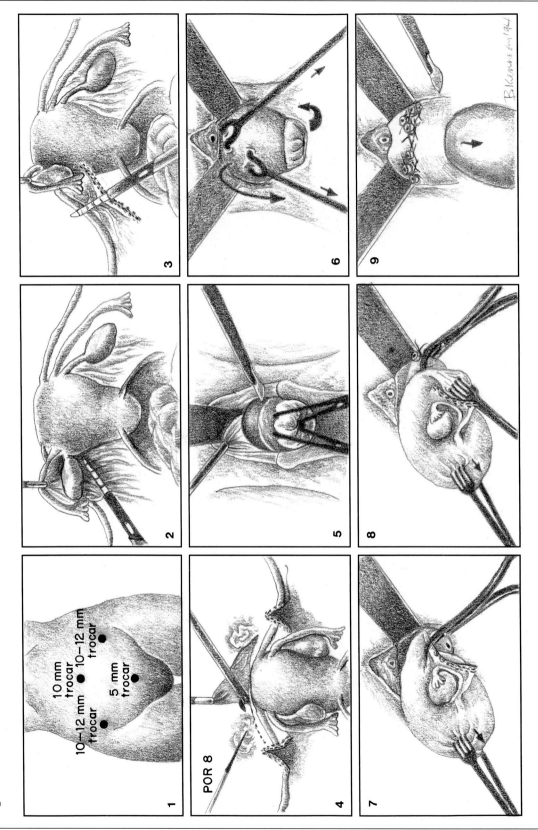

Figure 17.6

stapler below the uterine vessels may be risky.

The vaginal portion of the procedure is depicted in Fig. 17.6. The uterine fundus is delivered via an anterior colpotomy opening. This eliminates the necessity to perform a posterior colpotomy. The integrity of the posterior cul de sac is maintained and the risk of enterocele is reduced. After the vaginal cuff is closed, the operative field is inspected by laparoscope. This is done after the intra-abdominal pressure is decreased to 6 mmHg. Irrigation of the operative field and haemostasis if necessary are done.

Total laparoscopic assisted vaginal hysterectomy (TLAVH)

In TLAVH (Fig. 17.7), the round ligament is divided using a stapler incorporating the posterior broad ligament. If the adnexa is to be removed, the incision is extended to the broad ligament lateral to the adnexa, lateral and parallel to the infundibulopelvic ligament. The infundibulopelvic ligament is then skeletonized, stapled and transected. The ureters must always be identified and this can be achieved by opening the peritoneum above the pelvic brim or by dissecting the ureter on the pelvic sidewall. Alternatively, the peritoneum superior to the most distal part of the ureter is opened to approximately 1 cm. Dissection above this marked point is considered safe. The bladder is dissected off the cervix as in LAVH. In TLAVH, the uterine vessels are skeletonized, stapled and transected. Because of the close proximity of the vessels to the ureter, we recommend the use of mechanical devices such as stapler or clips.

Skeletonization, stapling and transection are continued on the cardinal ligaments until the uterosacral ligaments. As in LAVH, in order to apply the stapler parallel to and adjacent to the uterus, the laparoscope must be placed in the lower trocar and the stapler in the umbilical port.

A colpotomy incision is then made. The site of colpotomy is determined with the help of vaginal and rectal probes or a "colpotomizer". The remainder of the procedure can be completed vaginally or laparoscopically. At the completion of the operation, all pedicles are inspected by the laparoscope to ascertain that haemostasis is secured.

LAPAROSCOPIC SUBTOTAL (SUPRACERVICAL) HYSTERECTOMY

Subtotal or supracervical hysterectomy has recently regained its popularity. It has similar advantages to CISH, but the entire cervix is preserved. It is known that the risk of malignancy of the cervical stump in a woman who has had consecutive negative cervical cytology is very low. The incidence is equal to vaginal vault cancer (3–5 per 1000 women).

The procedure is initially done in a manner similar to other laparoscopic hysterectomies. However, after ligation of the uterine vessels, a pretied ligature (loop) is placed around the cervix (Fig. 17.8). The intrauterine cannula is removed and another loop is applied. The uterine corpus is separated from the cervix using scissors or a unipolar needle electrode (Fig. 17.9). The endocervix is coagulated and the uterus is removed with a morcellator (Fig. 17.10).

Figure 17.6 (opposite)   *Laparoscopic assisted vaginal hysterectomy:*
1. *Trocar sites.*
2. *Stapling the infundibulopelvic ligament.*
3. *Stapling the round ligament.*
4. *The development of the bladder flap.*
5. *Anterior colpotomy incision.*

6. *The fundus is delivered through an anterior colpotomy opening.*
7,8. *Clamp, cut and suture–ligate the uterine vessels, cardinal ligaments and the uterosacral ligaments.*
9. *Clamp the posterior cuff, cut the specimen and suture the posterior cuff.*

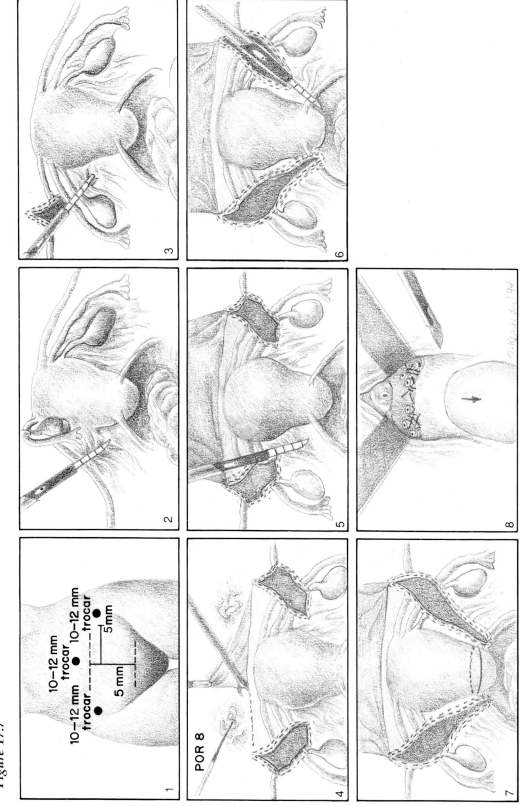

Figure 17.7

LAPAROSCOPIC TOTAL INTRAFASCIAL HYSTERECTOMY

Here, after ligature of the uterine vessels, the cervix is circumcized. This is done by incising the cervix circumferentially at the level of internal os preserving the uterosacral and the cardinal ligaments and the entire length of the vagina. The opening is closed with 0-Vicryl incorporating all the ligaments.

POTENTIAL COMPLICATIONS AND THEIR PREVENTION

CISH and IVH involve excision of the functional tissue of the cervix. The risk of developing malignancy from the remaining cervical muscle and connective tissue is extremely small.

1. Preoperative complication prevention. A preoperative examination and bowel prep on the day before the operation are important. The availability of basic surgical instruments and apparatus including instruments for haemostasis such as clips, ligatures, sutures or staplers is mandatory. The patient is always prepared for a laparotomy in such a way that conversion to laparotomy is not considered a complication but an extension of the procedure for a better treatment.

2. Postoperative complication prevention. Preoperatively, the patient should be warned about the possibility of complications including bowel perforation, ureteral injury and other possible complications of laparoscopy. In the postoperative period, observations of fever, urinary symptoms, abdominal distention, bowel habit and abdominal pain are extremely important. If a drain is used, the colour and quantity of the drainage fluid should be evaluated.

3. A special risk of CISH and subtotal hysterectomy is slippage of the loop around the cervical stump and bleeding from the ascending branch of the uterine arteries.

4. Ureteral injury. The course of the ureter should always be followed before and during the hysterectomy. The endoscopic stapler must be used cautiously.

Figure 17.7 (opposite) *Total laparoscopic assisted vaginal hysterectomy (TLAVH):*
1. *Trocar sites.*
2. *Stapling the round ligament.*
3. *Stapling the utero-ovarian ligament.*
4. *Injection of vasopressin derivative and development of the bladder flap.*
5. *Stapling of the cardinal ligament and uterine vessels.*
6. *Stapling and transection of the uterosacral ligament.*
7. *Anterior and posterior colpotomy incisions.*
8. *Vaginal extraction of the uterus.*

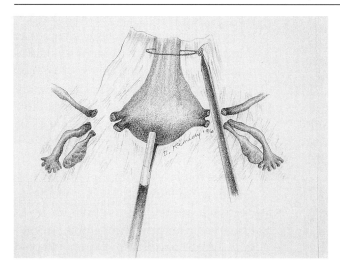

Figure 17.8 Laparoscopic subtotal hysterectomy: application of a pretied ligature (loop) after ligation of the uterine vessels.

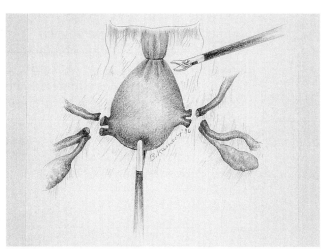

Figure 17.9 Separating the uterine corpus from the cervix.

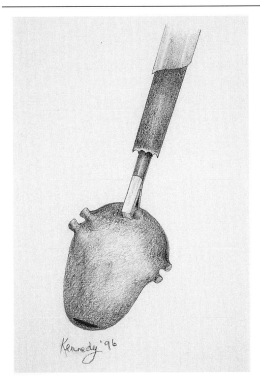

Figure 17.10 Morcellation of the uterine corpus.

SUGGESTED READING

Donnez J, Smets M, Polet R, Bassil S, Nissole M: LASH: laparoscopic supracervical (subtotal) hysterectomy. *Zentralbl Gynakol* 1995 **117**: 629–632.

Lee PI: Total laparoscopic intrafascial hysterectomy. *Gynaecol Endosc* 1997 **6**: 219–224.

Mettler L: Einsatz des Endo-Staplers (Multifire Endo GIA™ 30) zur endosckopisscheen Ovar, Adnex- oder Tubektomie sowie intrafaszialen Hysterektomie ohne Kolpotomie. *Minimal Invasive Chirurgie* 1993 **2**: 10–13.

Mettler L, Semm K, Lüttges JE, Panadikar D: Pelviskopische intrafasziale hysterectomie ohne Kolpotomie (CISH). *Gynekol Prax* 1993 **17**: 509–526.

Semm K: *Operationslehre fur endoskopische Abdominalchirurgie.* Schattauer, Stuttgart, New York, 1984.

Semm K: Hysterektomie per laparotomiam oder per pelviscopiam. Ein neuer Weg ohne Kolpotomie durch CASH. *Geburtsh Frauenheilk* 1991 **51**: 996–1003.

18

LAPAROSCOPIC RADICAL HYSTERECTOMY

Daniel S. Seidman, Camran Nezhat, Farr Nezhat, Ceana Nezhat

Laparoscopic surgery may offer important advantages to women undergoing radical hysterectomy. The low degree of postoperative pain, the rapid recovery, and the early postoperative ambulation typical for laparoscopic surgery, are of special benefit, as they reduce the need for analgesic drugs and the risk for paralytic ileus, and more importantly thromboembolic complications. Other advantages of laparoscopy, including lower incidence of infection and less adhesion formation, may also serve to encourage the use of laparoscopic surgery for young women with cervical cancer. One important factor in laparoscopic surgery is magnification. Thus, better exposure makes it ideal for performing radical hysterectomy endoscopically.

STAGES IN THE PROCEDURE

1. First, the upper abdomen and pelvis are inspected, steep Trendelenburg (30°) is obtained, and the bowel is displaced to the upper abdomen.
2. Para-aortic node dissection (if indicated) is performed and specimens are sent for frozen section. If the lymph nodes are negative, the operator proceeds with radical hysterectomy and pelvic node dissection. An assistant performs simultaneous rectal and vaginal examination, delineating the rectum and vagina.

3. The cul-de-sac is incised; the rectum is pushed from the posterior vaginal wall using CO_2 laser, electricity, blunt dissection, and hydrodissection to a level 4–5 cm below the cervix (Fig. 18.1).

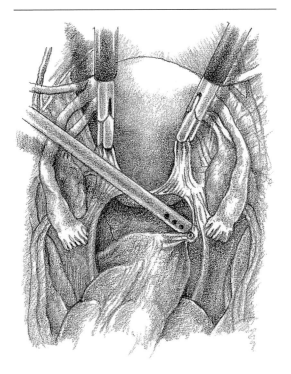

Figure 18.1 *Complete development of the rectovaginal space. Sharp dissection with the CO_2 laser, blunt dissection and hydrodissection are used.*

4. For the paravesical space, the line of dissection is between the round ligament anteriorly, infundibulopelvic ligament medially and pelvic side wall laterally (Fig. 18.2). The round ligaments (Fig. 18.3) are desiccated close to the pelvic side walls and transected. The peritoneum is opened and the obliterated hypogastric artery is identified and pulled medially and entered into the paravesical space between the pelvic side wall and the artery. Using sharp, blunt and hydrodissection, the obturator space is entered and the obturator nerve and vessels are identified; obliterated hypogastric artery skeletonized and traced down until ureter and branches of hypogastric artery are seen (Figs 18.4 and 18.5). Dissection continues inferiorly and the pararectal space developed. The uterine vessels are identified, skeletonized and electrodesiccated or clipped just medial to their origin and transected (Fig. 18.6). They are grasped with the forceps and rotated anterior to the ureters. This separation from the ureters must be gentle. Small blood vessels from the uterine artery to ureter are desiccated with bipolar forceps or clipped.

5. To develop the vesicovaginal space, the bladder peritoneum is injected with lactated Ringer's solution. The anterior leaf of the broad ligament is opened and the bladder flap is developed. After dividing scar tissue and the vesicouterine fold, the bladder is pushed completely from the cervix and upper vagina using the suction-irrigator probe (Fig. 18.7).

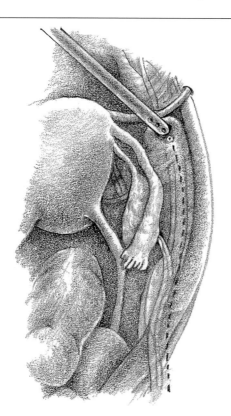

Figure 18.2 *The right paravesical space is developed by opening the peritoneum and performing hydrodissection. The line is between the round ligament anteriorly, infundibulopelvic ligament medially, and pelvic side wall laterally.*

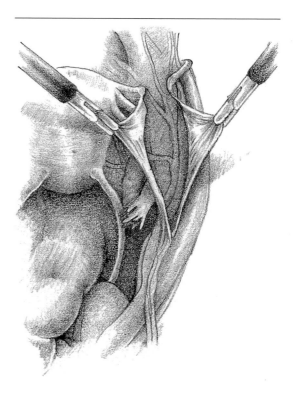

Figure 18.3 *After electrodesiccation and cutting the right round ligament, the peritoneum is grasped laterally and the paravesical space is exposed.*

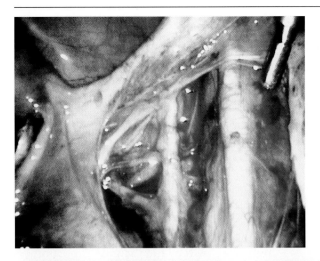

Figure 18.4 *Anatomy at radical hysterectomy. From the right: external iliac artery, hypogastric artery, uterine and superior vesical arteries originating from the hypogastric artery.*

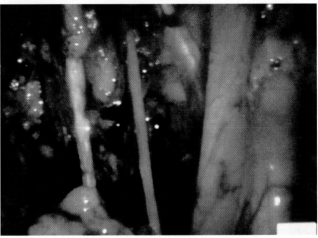

Figure 18.5 *Anatomy at radical hysterectomy. From the right: external iliac artery and vein, obturator nerve, bony pelvis, pelvic nodes.*

6. The utero-ovarian or infundibulopelvic pedicles are electrodesiccated with bipolar forceps and transected with scissors or laser. Alternatively, a laparoscopic stapling device can be used to achieve haemostasis and to cut large pedicles. The uterus is retracted medially and the direction of the ureter to the bladder and ureteral canal identified. Using gentle sharp and blunt dissection, the ureter is skeletonized to the bladder. The uterosacral ligaments and lateral parametria are stapled or desiccated with bipolar forceps and sequentially transected approximately 1.5–3 cm lateral to the cervix, based on the type of radical hysterectomy that has been performed. The dissection is taken to 2–3 cm below the cervix.

7. The vagina is entered anteriorly and posteriorly. A ring forceps attached to a 4×4 gauze or right-angle retractor is placed into the vagina to push its walls anteriorly and posteriorly, allowing it to be incised from above. To preserve pneumoperitoneum, two wet sponges are placed in a surgical glove and inserted into the vagina.

8. The procedure is completed laparoscopically by incising the vagina laparoscopically while the assistant identifies the vagina by placing a sponge forceps in it. Manipulation can be difficult, particularly if the uterus is enlarged, and it may be easier to complete the procedure vaginally, by incising the vagina 3 cm distal to the cervix. The residual cardinal

ligaments are mobilized then divided approximately 1.5–3 cm lateral to the cervix and suture ligated. After the uterus is removed, the vaginal cuff is left open until the lymph nodes are removed from the abdomen. Then, it is closed vaginally or laparoscopically with 0 Vicryl laparoscopic sutures.

Alternatively, the procedure is begun laparoscopically and completed vaginally. The laparoscopic portion includes development of the paravesical space, separation and ligation of the uterine vessels at their origin, medial displacement of the ureters and pelvic lymphadenectomy. The remainder of the operation is completed vaginally using a Schauta procedure, including dissection of the vagina, ureters and parametrium. After the vaginal portion is completed, laparoscopic evaluation is performed again. All pedicles and both ureters are evaluated and haemostasis is ensured under low pneumoperitoneal pressure. No drains are inserted, and the peritoneum is left open to allow lymph drainage into the peritoneal cavity and prevent lymphocyst formation. Suprapubic or transurethral catheters are removed after 1–2 weeks and routine bladder training is performed. Pelvic lymphadenectomy is performed at this stage. The technique is described in Chapter 19.

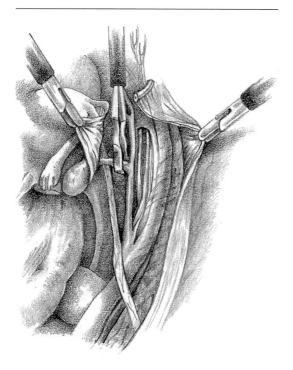

Figure 18.6 *The uterine artery is electrodesiccated at its origin from the hypogastric artery using bipolar forceps.*

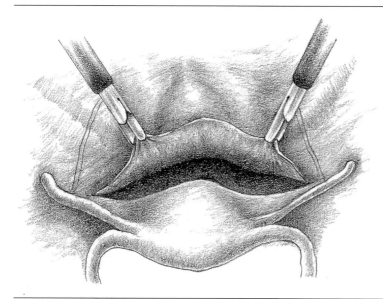

Figure 18.7 *Developing the vesicovaginal space. The anterior leaf of the broad ligament is elevated with grasping forceps and hydrodissection is performed.*

POTENTIAL COMPLICATIONS AND THEIR PREVENTION

The major postoperative complications of radical hysterectomy are bladder dysfunction, formation of ureteral fistulae, lymphocysts, pelvic infection and haemorrhage. All of these complications are considered preventable through improvement in techniques, such as avoiding excess damage to the ureter and preserving alternate routes of blood supply. The use of electrosurgery and haemoclips has been instrumental in assisting the surgeon with haemostasis, and minimizing postoperative haemorrhage. Operative mortality from radical hysterectomy has decreased from eight in 473 cases reported in 1955 to zero in some recent studies. Morbidity, as reflected by urinary fistula incidence, has decreased from more than 20% to less than 1%. The introduction of laparoscopic surgery has been viewed by some as the next step toward further reducing postoperative complications. The safety, adequacy, and apparent benefits of laparoscopic radical hysterectomy and lymphadenectomy have been clearly demonstrated. However, the precise future role of this surgical technique will be determined by prospective randomized trials.

SUGGESTED READING

Childers JM, Hatch K, Surwit EA: The role of laparoscopic lymphadenectomy in the management of cervical carcinoma. *Gynecol Oncol* 1992 **47**: 38–43.

Lee CL, Huang KG, Lai YM, Lai CH, Soong YK: Ureteral injury during laparoscopically assisted radical vaginal hysterectomy. *Hum Reprod* 1995 **10**: 2047–2049.

Mattingly RF, Thompson JD (eds): *Te Linde's Operative Gynecology*, 6th edn. JB Lippincott, Philadelphia, 1985, pp. 814.

Nezhat CR, Nezhat FR, Ramirez CE *et al.*: Laparoscopic radical hysterectomy and laparoscopic assisted vaginal radical hysterectomy with pelvic and paraaortic node dissection. *J Gynecol Surg* 1993 **9**: 105–120.

Querleu D: Laparoscopically assisted radical vaginal hysterectomy. *Gynecol Oncol* 1993 **51**: 248–254.

Schauta F: Die operation des gebarmutterkrebses mittels des schuchardt'schen aravaginalschnittes. *Montasschr Z Geburtschif Gynakol* 1902 **15**: 133.

19

LAPAROSCOPIC PELVIC AND AORTIC LYMPHADENECTOMY

Nicholas Kadar

Pelvic and aortic lymphadenectomy can be performed by laparoscopy and in experienced hands, they are associated with lower morbidity than by laparotomy. The adequacy of laparoscopic lymphadenectomy is determined by the number of lymph nodes removed, the proportion of patients found to have nodal disease and ultimately by the survival rates. Photographs of the completed dissection provide further objective indication of the extensiveness and limits of the dissection performed. Kadar appears to have been the first to perform complete pelvic lymphadenectomy as opposed to lymph node sampling by laparoscopy. This is a procedure that requires mobilization of the iliac vessels from the psoas muscle, separation of the iliac artery and vein and their "skeletonization". Right-sided aortic lymph node sampling was first performed by Childers and Surwit. Kadar and Spirtos appear to have been the first to perform left-sided aortic lymph node sampling and Kadar was the first to remove fixed, enlarged malignant para-aortic lymph nodes (both left and right sided).

PROCEDURE

The most important principle underlying the techniques for retroperitoneal dissection is that the peritoneum is the best bowel retractor. Peritoneal incisions are kept small, and no structure or ligament is divided until dissection of the retroperitoneum is complete.

Development of pelvic spaces and dissection of the ureter

These are done before pelvic lymphadenectomy. The steps in the procedures are as follows.

Step 1. Opening the pelvic side wall triangles

The triangle of the pelvic side wall is delineated by displacing the uterus to the contralateral side. The base of this triangle is formed by the round ligament, the lateral border by the external iliac artery, the medial border by the infundibulopelvic ligament, and the apex by where the infundibulopelvic ligament crosses the common iliac artery (Fig. 19.1). The peritoneum in the middle of the triangle is incised and the broad ligament opened by bluntly separating the extraperitoneal areolar tissues.

The peritoneal incision is extended first to the round ligament, which is not divided at this time, and then to the apex of the triangle, lateral to the infundibulopelvic ligament (Fig. 19.2). On the left side, so-called congenital adhesions attach the rectosigmoid to the peritoneum laterally, at or just above the pelvic brim. These usually cover the apex of the pelvic triangle. The dissection on the left side is begun by separating

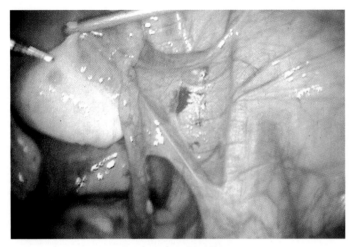

Figure 19.1 *The triangle of the pelvic side wall is formed by the round ligament, the lateral border by the external iliac artery and the medial border by the infundibulopelvic ligament. From Kadar N:* Atlas of Laparoscopic Pelvic Surgery. *Blackwell Scientific Publications, Oxford, 1994. Reproduced with permission.*

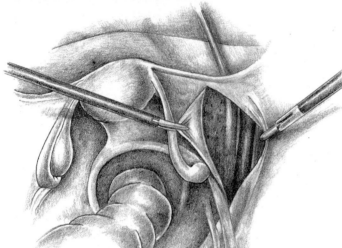

Figure 19.2 *The peritoneal incision is extended to the round ligament and then to the apex of the triangle lateral to the infundibulopelvic ligament. From Kadar N:* Atlas of Laparoscopic Pelvic Surgery. *Blackwell Scientific Publications, Oxford, 1994.*

these adhesions from the underlying peritoneum, and the pelvic side wall triangle is opened at or near its apex (Fig. 19.3). (The external iliac artery will be below the plane of dissection.) The peritoneal incision is then carried distally to the round ligament.

Step 2. Identification of the ureter at the apex of the pelvic triangle

The infundibulopelvic ligament is pulled medially with grasping forceps to expose the ureter at the pelvic brim where it crosses the common or external iliac artery (Fig. 19.4). It is crucial to mobilize the infundibulopelvic ligament adequately. This is done

by extending the peritoneal incision much further proximally, frequently to the caecum on the right, and the descending colon in the paracolic gutter on the left.

The dissection of the apex is more difficult on the left side partly because the ureter is covered by the mesentery of the sigmoid colon, but mainly because it crosses the iliac vessels higher (more proximally), and consequently lies more medial than the right ureter. The peritoneal incision has to be extended to the white line in the paracolic gutter to mobilize the sigmoid colon, and with it the infundibulopelvic ligament, which at this point lies extraperitoneally, under the mesentery (Fig. 19.5).

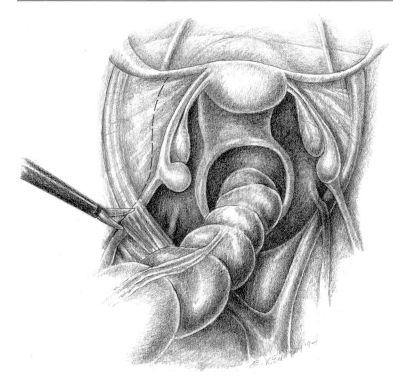

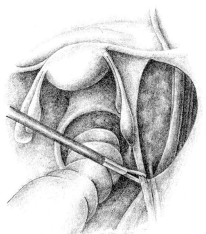

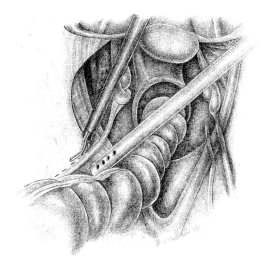

Figure 19.3 *The attachments of the sigmoid colon are divided and the incision on the left started at the apex of the triangle of the pelvic side wall triangle. From Kadar N:* Atlas of Laparoscopic Pelvic Surgery. *Blackwell Scientific Publications, Oxford, 1994.*

Figure 19.4 *The infundibulopelvic ligament is mobilized and pulled medially to expose the ureter at the pelvic brim. From Kadar N:* Atlas of Laparoscopic Pelvic Surgery. *Blackwell Scientific Publications, Oxford, 1994.*

Figure 19.5 *Mobilization of the left infundibulopelvic ligament. From Kadar N:* Atlas of Laparoscopic Pelvic Surgery. *Blackwell Scientific Publications, Oxford, 1994.*

*Step 3. Identification of the obliterated
hypogastric arteries extraperitoneally*

The dissection is carried bluntly underneath
and caudad to the round ligament, until the
obliterated hypogastric artery is identified
extraperitoneally (Fig. 19.6). If any difficulty
is encountered, the artery should be first
identified intraperitoneally where it hangs
from the anterior abdominal wall, then
traced proximally to where it passes behind
the round ligament.

Step 4. Development of paravesical spaces

The paravesical space is developed by
bluntly separating the areolar tissue on
either side of the external iliac artery. The
dissection is started lateral to the artery,
mindful that the external iliac vein is just
lateral to it. The tips of the closed dissecting
scissors are placed against the lateral edge
of the artery and the artery is pulled medially, whereupon a bloodless plane will open
lateral to it (Fig. 19.7). The medial border of
the artery is then freed in an identical manner, but working in the opposite direction.
During this manoeuvre the operator must
take care not to press on the external iliac
vein as the artery is displaced laterally (Fig.
19.8). For a hysterectomy and pelvic
lymphadenectomy, the paracervical spaces
should be developed adequately to obtain
good exposure of the uterine arteries and
cardinal ligaments distally. This provides
complete control of the operative field,
especially if the arteries bleed when they are
divided, which can occur despite what
appears to be adequate bipolar desiccation.

Step 5. Development of pararectal spaces

The obliterated hypogastric arteries are next
traced proximally to where they are joined
by the uterine arteries, and the pararectal
spaces opened by blunt dissection proximal
and medial to the uterine vessels, which lie
on top of the cardinal ligaments. Once the
pararectal spaces have been opened, the
ureter on the ipsilateral side is easily identified on the medial leaf of the broad ligament, which forms the medial border of the
pararectal space. The uterine artery and cardinal ligament at the distal (caudal) border
of the space, and the internal iliac artery on
its lateral border also become clearly visible
at this stage (Figs 19.9 and 19.10). The uterine artery can easily be ligated.

Laparoscopic pelvic lymphadenectomy

Laparoscopic pelvic lymphadenectomy is
done in exactly the same way as the open
operation. Indeed, the surgeon will obtain a

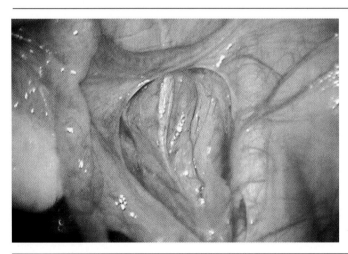

Figure 19.6 *The extraperitoneal
portion of the obliterated hypogastric
artery is identified. From Kadar N:*
Atlas of Laparoscopic Pelvic
Surgery, *Blackwell Scientific
Publications, Oxford, 1994.*

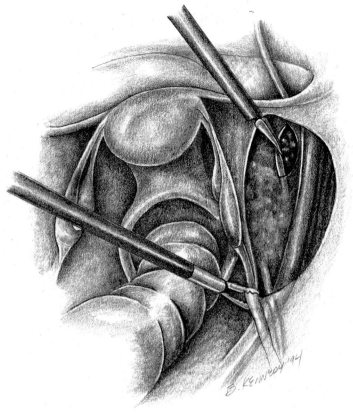

Figure 19.7 *The lateral paravesical space is opened. From Kadar N:* Atlas of Laparoscopic Pelvic Surgery. *Blackwell Scientific Publications, Oxford, 1994.*

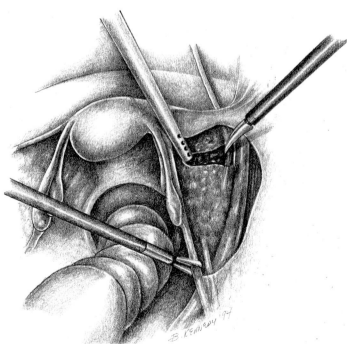

Figure 19.8 *The medial paravesical space is opened. From Kadar N:* Atlas of Laparoscopic Pelvic Surgery. *Blackwell Scientific Publications, Oxford, 1994.*

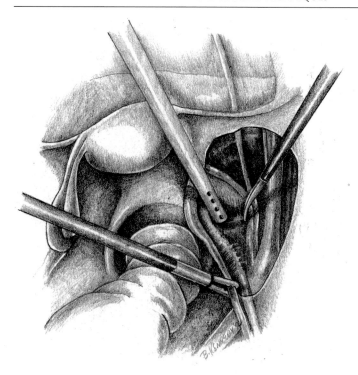

Figure 19.9 *The pararectal space is developed; the ureter lies on its medial border.*

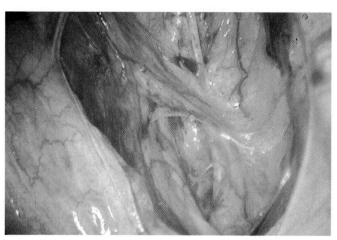

Figure 19.10 *All anatomical structures involved are demonstrated. The uterine artery is seen crossing the right ureter after its origin from the hypogastric artery.*

better view of the obturator fossa than at laparotomy. The pelvic spaces are first developed and ureters identified as described above. The surgical limits of the dissection are then delineated. These are the common iliac artery proximally (i.e. cephalad), the psoas muscle laterally, the circumflex iliac vein and pubic bone distally (i.e. caudad), the obliterated umbilical artery medially, and the obturator fossa inferiorly

(i.e. ventrally). The sequence of the operation is as follows.

Step 1. Mobilization of external iliac vessels from the psoas muscle and entry into the obturator fossa lateral to the vessels (Fig. 19.11)

To mobilize the external iliac vessels, the dense areolar tissue attaching the vessels to the psoas muscle is incised very superfi-

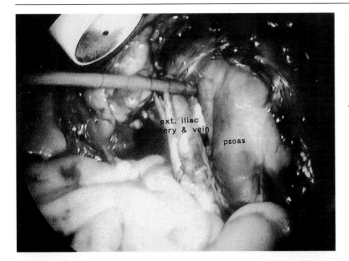

Figure 19.11 Laparoscopic pelvic lymphadenectomy. Nodal tissue has been removed from in front of the psoas muscle and external iliac artery, and the external vessels are being mobilized from the psoas muscle.

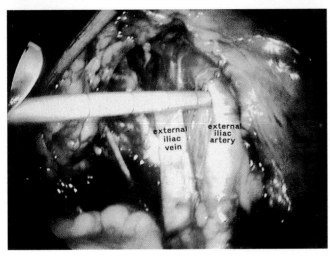

Figure 19.12 The areolar sheaths around the external iliac vessels have been removed and the vessels separated.

cially from the common iliac artery to the circumflex iliac vein. Using blunt dissection, the external iliac artery and vein are peeled off the psoas muscle. Once the vein is freed, with progressively deeper dissection the surgeon will gain entry into the obturator fossa. This is identified by the bright yellow fatty-nodal tissue that comes into view.

Step 2. Liberation of the external iliac artery and vein from the surrounding areolar sheath and separation of the vessels (Fig. 19.12)

The external iliac artery and vein are completely surrounded by their own distinct areolar sheath, and the two sheaths are fused along the entire course of the vessels. The sheath of the external iliac artery is incised with scissors along its dorsal surface from the level of the common iliac artery down to the circumflex iliac vein. At this point, the sheaths of the external iliac artery and vein are still joined along the undersurface of the artery. The next step is to incise the sheath of the external iliac vein. This has to be done with utmost care. In order to gain access to the obturator fossa, the inferior border of the vein which is tethered by loose areolar tissue to the pelvic side wall and obturator fossa is freed.

Step 3. Removal of fatty-node bearing tissue from the front of the psoas muscle and the external iliac vessels

The fatty-nodal tissue in front of the psoas muscle and external iliac vessels is removed by grasping the tissue with a spoon forceps and freeing its areolar attachments with sharp scissor dissection. The most lateral part of this nodal bundle is about 2–3 cm from the artery itself, and has a nutrient branch that has to be coagulated as these nodes are freed from the inferolateral part of the psoas muscle. The medial attachments of these nodes are freed when the external iliac vessels are dissected from their sheaths. Accordingly, all that remains is to free their lateral attachments to the psoas muscle. As this is done, the iliofemoral and genito-femoral nerves are encountered and these can easily be pushed laterally.

Step 4. Freeing the obturator nerve from the fatty-nodal bundle in the obturator fossa and dissection of the obturator nodes from the pubic bone and the internal iliac artery until the bifurcation of the iliac artery

Finally, the obturator fossa and internal iliac vessels are freed. This is done by retracting the external iliac vessels laterally, and teasing out the obturator nerve from the most inferior part of the obturator nodal bundle. Once the nerve is freed, the distal attachments of the nodal bundle can be freed from the pubic bone by dividing them with a cutting current to seal the lymphatics. The nodal bundle is grasped and removed. Eventually, the internal iliac artery is reached, and the nodal tissue lying anterior, lateral and medial to it is freed in continuity with the obturator fossa nodal mass. The nodal tissue can be quite adherent in this region because the internal iliac artery does not have an areolar sheath as do the external iliac vessels.

Step 5. Retraction of the external iliac vein laterally to ensure that the bifurcation of the iliac artery has been completely cleared of node bearing tissue

Any nodal tissue lying lateral to and in front of the lower part of the common iliac artery is also freed at this point. With further dissection in a cephalad direction, the crura or bifurcation of the iliac arteries is reached. Note that the external and internal iliac veins lie just lateral to these structures. Once the attachments of the nodal bundle in this region are divided, the dissection is complete (Fig. 19.13).

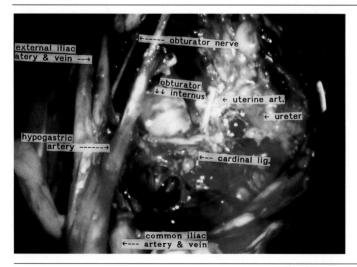

Figure 19.13 *Completed laparoscopic pelvic lymphadenectomy in a patient with stage IBII carcinoma of the cervix undergoing laparo-vaginal radical hysterectomy.*

Laparoscopic aortic lymphadenectomy

After a pneumoperitoneum is established and the trocars inserted, the patient is positioned in steep Trendelenburg position and rotated slightly to her left. The abdomen and pelvis are inspected, and peritoneal washings are taken. The laparoscope is switched to the suprapubic port, and the video monitors are positioned at the head of the table as for a cholecystectomy. The surgeon stands on the patient's right side. Standing between the patient's legs gives a natural anatomical view of the retroperitoneum, but it makes camera manipulation awkward. The sigmoid colon is displaced laterally with the rectal probe, small bowel displaced from the pelvis, and the root of the mesentery elevated.

Peritoneal incision

The easiest and most natural posterior peritoneal incision is over the right common iliac artery, parallel to the root of the small bowel mesentery from the caecum to the ligament of Treitz. Although initially it is more difficult to identify the retroperitoneal structures, we prefer to enter the retroperitoneum through a small incision in the posterior parietal peritoneum placed directly in front of the aorta (pre-aortic incision). If difficulty is encountered in keeping the small bowel out of the way, a more distal site is selected, just above the sacral promontory, medial to the sigmoid mesentery. Once the peritoneum has been incised it can be elevated and used to keep bowel out of the way.

Planes of dissection

The peritoneal incision is extended proximally to the root of the small bowel mesentery, and distally to a point in front of or cephalad to the sacral promontory. The incision is extended gradually. Using blunt dissection, a plane is developed between the peritoneum and the node bearing fatty areolar tissue overlying the great vessels. The plane is extended laterally on each side to the ureters, which are elevated with the peritoneum. On the left, the dissection is performed under the inferior mesenteric artery, which is elevated with the mesentery of the descending colon. Once the correct plane has been developed, the duodenum is elevated by blunt dissection with the suction irrigator or a probe.

The node bearing areolar tissue in front of the aorta is incised and the incision is carried down to the adventitia of the aorta. It is not always easy to know where to make this incision because the great vessels are covered by node bearing tissue and the aorta can usually only be seen clearly in thin patients without retroperitoneal pathology. The duodenum and the origin of the inferior mesenteric artery are also usually ill-defined. However, it is usually possible to "feel" the sacrum with a dissecting probe, which serves as a useful guide to the midline. The pulsations of the aorta can often be "felt" if it is gently pressed with a probe, but much less clearly than one might imagine.

The nodal tissue is incised high just below the inferior mesenteric artery and below the inferior leaf of the small bowel mesentery (Fig. 19.14). If the dissection is started too low there is a danger of injuring the left common iliac vein as it crosses the midline below the bifurcation of the aorta, above the sacral promontory. Once the plane between the aorta and the overlying nodal tissue has been developed and the glistening surface of the aorta is seen, the dissection is straight forward. The biggest challenge is to keep bowel out of the way. This is done by elevating the posterior parietal peritoneum, and the peritoneal incision should be kept small.

Removal of the fatty-nodal tissue; lymphadenectomy proper

The limits of the dissection are the bifurcation of the aorta inferiorly and the ureters laterally. The superior extent of the dissection is either the third part of the duodenum

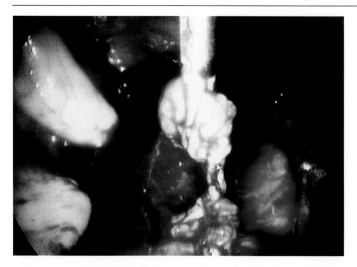

Figure 19.14 *Fixed, enlarged aortic lymph nodes removed from behind the inferior mesenteric artery.*

or the renal vein, in which case the duodenum must be mobilized. The nodal tissue is removed in systematic fashion. Working in a broad plane, the nodal tissue is mobilized "en bloc" from the front of the aorta and the upper part of the left common iliac artery, and extended as far laterally as possible. The nodal bundle is transected either proximally or distally, wherever it is most free (usually in front of the common iliac artery), and the tissue teased off the psoas, pushing the wall of the aorta somewhat medially. One needs to take care not to injure the vertebral arteries, and on no account pull hard if resistance to the dissection is encountered. If these arteries are injured and retract into the vertebral foramina, laparotomy will be necessary, and even then haemostasis may be difficult to secure.

The problem on the right side stems from the inability to see the wall of the inferior vena cava clearly until its areolar sheath has been incised. The wall of the vein merges imperceptibly with the investing tissue placing it at risk of injury during the initial incision into the sheath. The nodal tissue can then be grasped very superficially and elevated. Cautious dissection below the elevated tissue will allow one to enter the caval sheath. Once the glistening surface of the cava is seen the incision is extended proximally to the duodenum and inferiorly to the level of the right common iliac artery. The dissection is continued laterally along the psoas muscle as far as the right ureter. There are usually some small branches from the lower part of the vena cava which should be clipped or coagulated, although avulsion rather than division of the uncoagulated vessels is the major risk to guard against.

Dissection to the left renal vein is usually simple. Blunt dissection is used almost exclusively, and the duodenum elevated towards the right using the bowel graspers in the left upper and left lower trocars. The plane of dissection above the inferior mesenteric artery continues along the front of the aorta, towards the renal vein (Fig. 19.15). The ovarian artery is the first structure to be encountered, and has to be ligated. As the dissection continues to the left of the aorta and nodal tissue cleared from the front of the psoas muscle, the left ovarian vein is seen medial to the left ureter. It does not need to be ligated. On the right side, the right ovarian artery that crosses in front of the vena cava, and the right ovarian vein that drains into the front (or sometimes the side) of the vena cava have to be divided as node-bearing tissue lying lateral to and in front of the vena cava is removed. Nodal tissue between the aorta and vena cava is only removed after the adventitia of both the aorta and vena cava have been identified and are clearly visible (Fig. 19.16). The planes of dissection are extended up as far

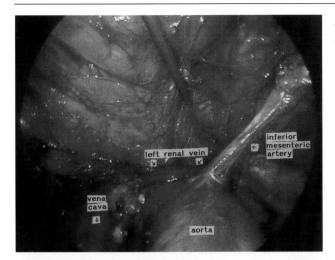

Figure 19.15 *Supramesenteric aortic lymphadenectomy.*

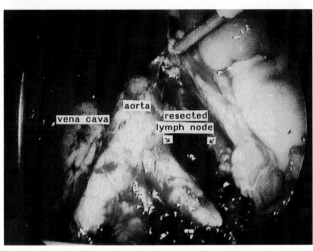

Figure 19.16 *Bilateral, laparoscopic inframesenteric aortic lymphadenectomy in a patient with stage IIIB cancer of the cervix. The "bed" of a large 50-mm lymph node containing metastatic disease can be seen to the left of the lower aorta.*

as the left renal vein, which is cleared of fatty-areolar tissue.

SUGGESTED READING

Childers JA, Surwit EA: Current status of operative laparoscopy in gynecologic oncology. *Oncology* 1993 **7**: 47–51.

Kadar N: Laparoscopic pelvic lymphadenectomy for the treatment of gynecological malignancies: description of a technique. *Gynecol Endosc* 1992 **1**: 79–83.

Kadar N: Laparoscopic resection of fixed and enlarged aortic lymph nodes in patients with advanced cervix cancer. *Gynecol Endosc* 1993 **2**: 217–221.

Kadar N: Laparoscopic radical vaginal hysterectomy: an operative technique and its evolution. *Gynecol Endosc* 1994 **3**: 109–122

Kadar N: Laparoscopic surgery for gynecologic malignancies in women aged 65 years or more. *Gynecol Endosc* 1995 **4**: 173–176.

Kadar N: Laparoscopic pelvic lymphadenectomy in obese women with gynecologic malignancies. *J Am Assoc Gynecol Laparosc* 1995 **2**: 81–85.

20

LAPAROSCOPIC TREATMENT OF URINARY STRESS INCONTINENCE

Thomas L. Lyons and Wendy K. Winer

Urinary stress incontinence and disorders of pelvic relaxation are an increasingly common problem encountered by gynecologists. Over 10 billion dollars were spent in the United States in 1988 on incontinence of which the greatest proportion was on urinary stress incontinence (USI). As the generation is getting older and yet remains physically active, it must be assumed that this number would have at least doubled in the last decade.

Understanding of the mechanisms involved in the female continence mechanism has improved in the last several years but it remains debatable. Some of the older methods of surgical correction for USI (anterior colporraphy and needle procedures) have not produced favourable long-lasting results whereas procedures such as the Burch procedure and the paravaginal repair have resulted in a more superior long-term outcome. Laparoscopic procedures have been directed toward replication of these superior techniques with decreased morbidity.

PATIENT SELECTION

Patients should be evaluated thoroughly before performing surgery for USI. History should include a detailed voiding diary, medication list, endocrinological history, and previous medical and surgical treatment.

Emphasis should be placed on eliciting symptoms suggesting detrusor dyssynergia or neurological pathology. Physical examination should include a full gynaecological examination and clinical urodynamic testing. Depending on the patient's presenting complaints and the results of physical examination, the urodynamic testings may include simple cystometrics and voiding evaluation or more complex multichannel urodynamics with urethral pressure profile or abdominal leak point pressure. The latter tests are performed to detect an intrinsic sphincter deficiency (ISD). ISD is more common in women over 65 years of age or in those individuals who have had multiple procedures for stress incontinence. Patients with ISD and a mobile anterior wall may be candidates for a suburethral sling procedure or if the anterior wall mobility is absent intraluminal bulking agents may be indicated. We have been successful in patients with anterior wall mobility and ISD using Burch/paravaginal repair plus bulking agents. This is a relatively low morbidity treatment with acceptable clinical results.

It seems that clinical evaluation correlates well with multichannel urodynamics (88+%). Accordingly, in patients with uncomplicated history and physical examination, we have used the following protocol.

- History: voiding diary, pharmaceutical regimen, endocrinopathy, prior gynecological or neurological surgery.

- Physical examination: general physical and gynecological examination, neurological evaluation of S2–S4, muscle tone and trigger points, full bladder examination in the lithotomy position, Valsalva or cough tests (Q-tip test), Marshall's or Bonney's maneuvre with Valsalva, timed void, urinalysis, and urine culture. Careful descriptive documentation of fascial defects are documented.
- Patients with confusing history or physical examination are submitted to more extensive testing.

TECHNICAL CONSIDERATIONS

There are over 100 operations described for the treatment of USI. These operations fall into one of three categories: vaginal repairs, needle procedures, and retropubic approaches. Among these, retropubic colposuspension (the Burch procedure) is considered the gold standard. It is important to emphasize that a global approach to defects in the pelvic floor produces superior results and that the first repair is the procedure most likely to succeed. For the above reasons it is important to examine the various types of procedures, the success rates, and the techniques described to accomplish these procedures laparoscopically.

Vaginal procedures such as anterior colporraphy with Kelly/Kennedy plication have been described as treatment for stress incontinence. The best data available suggest that it is successful in 50% of cases at one year follow-up. The vaginal approach to paravaginal repair is associated with good clinical and anatomical results. However, during the dissection, the perineal nerve could be affected leading to continued incontinence. This could occur also after the needle procedure. The ability to accomplish this procedure by laparoscopy without traumatic dissection makes it a logical alternative.

An abdominal approach to paravaginal repair with or without the Burch procedure is also effective. The laparoscopic efforts must therefore be attempted to replicate these established procedures while maintaining low morbidity. If clinical equivalency can be demonstrated with lower morbidity then the technique is viable.

Other procedures such as the Ball–Burch procedure and the suburethral sling can be accomplished laparoscopically and play defined roles in the care of patients with genuine stress incontinence and intrinsic sphincter deficiency.

PROCEDURE

The laparoscopic approach to the space of Retzius is accomplished by either the preperitoneal approach or the transperitoneal approach.

Preperitoneal approach

The preperitoneal approach begins by making an incision in the subumbilical area and opening the anterior leaf of the rectus fascia. The space can be dissected using a balloon apparatus, an optical trocar, or by simply allowing the pneumoperitoneum to open the space and using blunt dissection through the instrument channel of an operating laparoscope. It should be noted that this approach may be very difficult when the patient has had prior lower abdominal surgery. Because expansion of the anterior abdominal wall will compromise vision, if the patient requires posterior supportive procedure or a concomitant intra-abdominal procedure, the intra-abdominal work should be performed first. Secondary cannulas of 10 mm midline suprapubic (four fingerbreadths above the symphysis) and 5 mm just lateral to the left rectus muscle are placed after the space is opened under direct vision (Fig. 20.1a).

Transperitoneal approach

Here, the secondary trocars are a 10-mm trocar in the midline suprapubic, and two 5-mm ports lateral to the rectus muscles. These trocars are placed four fingerbreadths above the symphysis with good

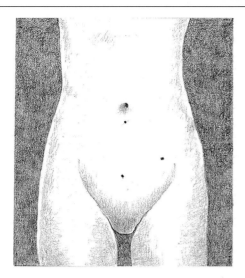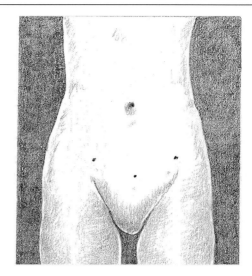

Figure 20.1 *Trocar sites for pre-peritoneal (left) and transperitoneal (right) approaches to the space of Retzius.*

separation necessary for suturing (Fig. 20.1b).

The transperitoneal approach is begun by identifying the pubic symphysis and making an incision in the anterior peritoneum approximately 1 inch (2.5 cm) above the symphysis. Be sure to make the incision well above the bladder. In women who have had surgery, the bladder can be located higher than its normal site. This incision is extended bilaterally through the obliterated umbilical ligaments and the space of Retzius is dissected bluntly.

The Cooper's ligaments are identified and cleaned of fat and areolar tissue. The lateral limits of the dissection is the obturator foramen, the obturator vascular bundle, the ischial spines, and the aberrant vasculature crossing the Cooper's ligament. The archus tendineous is seen extending from the ischial spine to the pubis. The paravaginal defects are dissected. The endopelvic fascia is cleaned of fat and the bladder is mobilized cephalad by placing fingers in the vagina and using a blunt dissector over these digits to move the bladder upward. After this preparation is completed, the operative field is clear and the anatomy reviewed for the reconstructive procedure

(Fig. 20.2).

The paravaginal defects should first be repaired using a figure of eight with 2-0 permanent suture starting at the ischial spine side of the defect (Fig. 20.3). Paraurethral vasculature can be encountered in this area but bleeding will usually subside as the sutures are tied. The size of the defect will dictate the number of sutures needed for closure. This repair will correct most cystoceles caused by lateral separation from archus tendineous attachment. Deep transverse defects of the pubocervical fascia must be repaired transabdominally and midline breaks in the vaginal endopelvic fascia (the rarest of the anterior vaginal defects) are repaired vaginally.

Two Burch sutures are then placed 1–2 cm lateral to the urethra (Fig. 20.4–20.7). These sutures are size 0 braided permanent suture. We use Ethibond™ (Ethicon, Inc. Sommerville, NJ). The first is placed at the midurethral level and the second at the urethrovesical junction. Both lower sutures are placed and tied and then the urethrovesical (U-V) junction sutures are placed and tied. If a single Burch suture is to be used, it should be placed at the U-V junction on each side. These sutures should not be

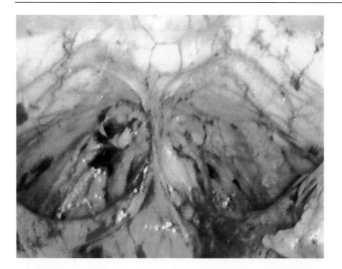

Figure 20.2 *The anatomy of the space of Retzius is reviewed before commencing the reconstructive procedure.*

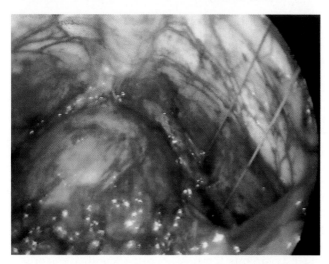

Figure 20.3 *Repairing the paravaginal defect using a 2-0 permanent suture material.*

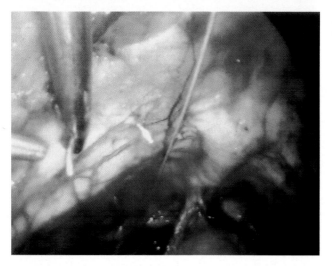

Figure 20.4 *Placing suture through Cooper's ligament.*

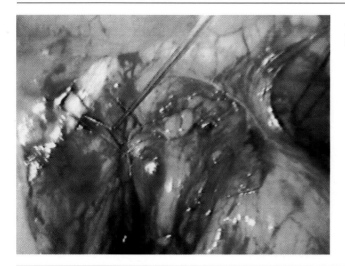

Figure 20.5 The sutures have been placed on each sides of the urethra.

tied tightly to Cooper's ligament. The goal is only to fixate the fascia and to create the "hammock" effect (Figs 20.6 and 20.7).

Other procedures

There are variations of the traditional Burch procedure. These include the use of a permanent mesh to attach the endopelvic fascia to Cooper's ligament (Ou *et al.*, 1993) and the use of an endoscopic stapler to attach the Burch sutures to Cooper's ligament (Lyons, 1995). Others have reported laparoscopic variations of the needle procedure. All of these are intended to make the procedure technically less demanding and they may well be the procedures of the future. But until long-term data are obtained they cannot be compared to the conventional procedures such as the classic laparoscopic Burch.

Posterior pelvic floor abnormalities should be corrected at the initiation of the procedure. Also, a McCall culdoplasty should be performed in all cases of Burch procedure to prevent the occurrence of enterocele. As stated earlier, a global approach to the pelvic floor is the most effective.

COMPLICATIONS AND THEIR PREVENTION

1. Surgical complications are similar to those associated with any laparoscopic procedure including bleeding and infection.
2. Urinary tract damage can occur but these problems can be diagnosed and managed at the time of surgery. Ureterolysis is routinely done before treatment of the posterior floor and cystoscopy is performed at the termination of each procedure. This is to evaluate ureteral integrity as well as to inspect the bladder for possible suture material.
3. Enterocele and rectocele are common following colposuspension and should be repaired during the primary surgery.
4. Voiding disorders are common but are transient.
5. A *de novo* rate of 17% detrusor dyssynergia is expected and can be treated with a combination of medical therapy and bladder training exercises. In our clinic, the drug of choice for this treatment is imipramine 25 mg once or twice daily. This agent has few side effects and is well tolerated by the older population who are more likely to have this problem.

CONCLUSION

After appropriate work-up and documentation for the need for surgical correction of USI, the physician can select a

Figure 20.6

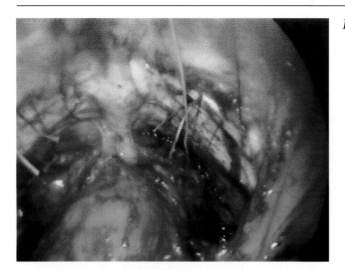

Figure 20.7

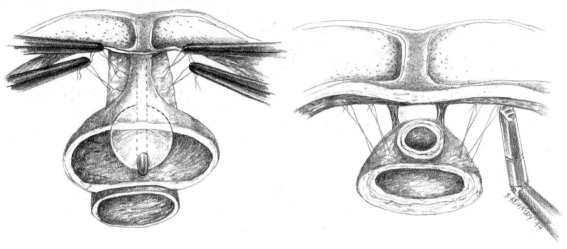

Figures 20.6 and 20.7 *The sutures should not be tied tightly to the Cooper's ligament. A "hammock" effect can be seen.*

minimally invasive approach that can reproduce the efficacy of traditional procedures while providing the reduced morbidity of laparoscopic surgery. At first the technical demands of this surgery seem prodigious but after laparoscopic suturing skills are obtained, the surgeon can perform these procedures easily and possibly with greater accuracy. The ability to visualize the defects of the pelvic floor *in vivo* by laparoscopy may contribute to our understanding of the pathophysiology of these disorders and to the success of the corrective procedures. Pelvic floor reconstruction remains a "work in progress" and continued understanding and improvement in surgical techniques is expected in the ensuing years.

SUGGESTED READING

Bergman A, Elia G: Three surgical procedures for genuine stress incontinence: five year follow-up of a prospective randomized study. *Am J Obstet Gynecol* 1995 **173**: 66–71.

Liu CY: Laparoscopic retropubic colposuspension. *Gynecol Endosc* 1993 **2**: 2.

Lyons TL: Minimally invasive treatment of urinary stress incontinence and laparoscopically directed repair of pelvic floor defects. *Clin Obstet Gynecol* 1995 **38**: 380.

Ou CS, Presthius J, Beadle E: Laparoscopic bladder neck suspension using hernia mesh. *Proceedings of the World Congress of Gynecologic Endoscopy, 22nd Annual Meeting of the American Association of Gynaecologic Laparoscopists*, 1993.

Vancaille TG, Schuessler W: Laparoscopic bladder neck suspension. *J Laparosc Endosc Surg* 1993 **1**: 169–173.

21

APPENDECTOMY

Togas Tulandi

Routine incidental appendectomy at the time of other abdominal or gynecological operations has been shown to be safe without increase in morbidity. The implications of its conduct during a laparoscopic surgery remain unclear. However, if during a laparoscopy examination, an inflamed appendix or appendiceal endometriosis is found, an appendectomy should be done.

PROCEDURE

The appendix is grasped with grasping forceps and gently stretched. If adhesion is encountered, this has to be dissected first. Using a bipolar cautery, the mesoappendix is coagulated approximately 1 cm beyond the base of the appendix (Fig. 21.1) and then divided (Fig. 21.2). Alternatively, the appendiceal vessels can be secured with staples. A pretied ligature (Endoloops, Rx Ethicon Inc., Sommerville, NJ; PercLoop, Laparomed, Irvine, CA) is applied around the base of the appendix, is tightened and cut (Figs 21.3 and 21.4). A second ligature is placed close and distal to the first and a third ligature is placed approximately 1 cm from the second. The appendix is transected with scissors between the second and the third loop (Fig.

21.5) and then removed from the abdominal cavity via a 10-mm portal. The appendiceal stump can be coagulated lightly with bipolar coagulation or vaporized with laser. Irrigation of the abdominal cavity is carefully done.

POTENTIAL COMPLICATIONS AND THEIR PREVENTION

1. Leakage from the stump: make sure that the loops are tight. Transecting the appendix with electrocautery may lead to breakage or loosening of the endoloops.
2. Bleeding: good haemostasis.
3. Caecal perforation due to heat damage.
4. Abscess.

CONTRAINDICATION

Contraindications to laparoscopic appendectomy include patients who are unstable, patients with Crohn's disease and patients undergoing radiotherapy. A walled-off perforated appendix is also better approached by laparotomy. Because an appendiceal mucocele can be malignant, a laparotomy by a general surgeon is indicated at another setting.

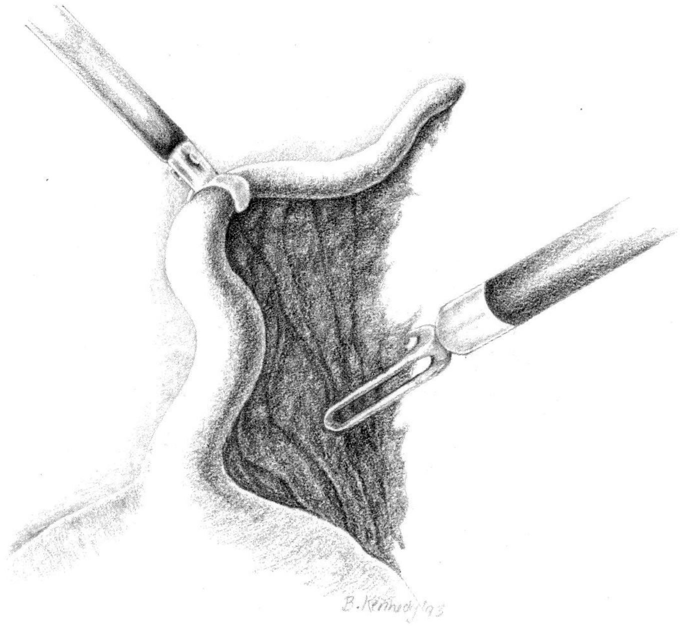

Figure 21.1

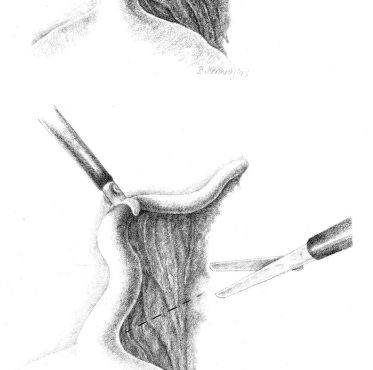

Figure 21.2

Figures 21.1 and 21.2
Coagulation and cutting of mesoappendix approximately 1 cm beyond the base of the appendix.

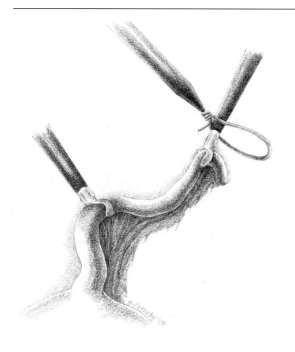

Figure 21.3

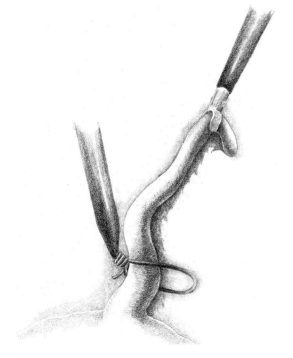

Figure 21.4

Figures 21.3 and 21.4 *Placement of a pretied ligature.*

Figure 21.5a

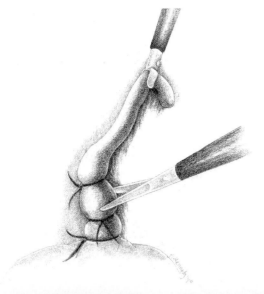

Figure 21.5b

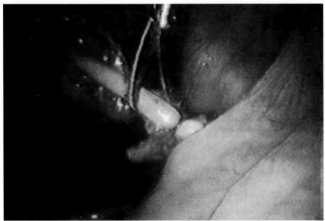

Figures 21.5a and 21.5b *Transection
of the appendix between the second
and the third ligatures.*

SUGGESTED READING

Pier A, Gotz F, Bacher C, Thevissen P: Laparoscopic appendectomy in 625 cases: from inno-
vation to routine. *Surg Laparosc Endosc* 1991 **1**:
8–13.

Richards W, Watson D, Lynch G, Reed GW,
Olsen D, Spaw A, Holcomb W, Frexes-Steed
M, Goldstein R, Sharp K: A review of the
results of laparoscopic versus open appendectomy. *Surg Gynecol Obstet* 1993 **177**:
473–480.

22

LAPAROSCOPIC TREATMENT OF UTERINE PROLAPSE

Arnaud Wattiez, Reinaldo Goldchmit, Michel Canis, Gerard Mage, Jean Luc Pouly and Maurice Antoine Bruhat

Fixation of the vaginal wall to the sacral promontory is called promontofixation. It was first introduced by Freund in 1889 but it was Otto Kustner in 1890 who used the technique to treat uterine prolapse in menopausal women. In 1958, Huguier and Scali reported promontofixation by laparotomy using Mersilene tape and subsequently in 1974, Scali *et al.* described a modified technique consisting of an anterior component providing subvesical support and a posterior component assisting promontofixation. Several authors have also described sacral-colpopexy by laparotomy as well as by laparoscopy. We performed our first laparoscopic promontofixation in 1991. Our technique offers the advantages for both abdominal and vaginal approaches by correcting uterine prolapse, treating stress incontinence and repairing cystocele or rectocele.

POSITIONING OF THE PATIENT

The usual laparoscopic positioning with the patient on her back and the legs abducted provides easy vaginal access. The buttocks are positioned close to the edge of the table facilitating uterine manipulation. A number 18 indwelling Foley catheter is inserted into the bladder. The balloon is inflated and is pulled back as far as possible to help identification of the bladder neck. The surgeon stands on the patient's left, the first assistant

on the right and the second assistant between the legs to provide uterine, vaginal and rectal manipulation.

PLACEMENT OF TROCARS

Four trocars are used: a 10-mm umbilical trocar for the laparoscope; another 10-mm trocar on the mid-low abdomen for introduction of needles and mesh; and two 5-mm trocars lateral to the inferior epigastric vessels (3 cm medial of the anterior superior iliac spines). The lower 10-mm trocar should not be placed lower than the two lateral ports. If the distance between the lower 10-mm trocar is less than 8 cm from the umbilicus, the umbilical trocar will be used for instrumentation and another 10-mm trocar will be placed above the umbilicus on the midline for the laparoscope.

TECHNIQUE

The steps involved in the laparoscopic treatment of uterine prolapse include:

1. Preparation of the vesicouterine and the vesicovaginal spaces;
2. Dissection of the broad ligament;
3. Posterior dissection;
4. Preparation of the promontory;
5. Fixation of the mesh in the vesicovaginal space;
6. Anterior reperitonealization;

7. Posterior reperitonealization;
8. Promontofixation;
9. Burch colposuspension.

Preparation of the vesicouterine and the vesicovaginal spaces

The dissection begins with the first assistant applying grasping forceps to the peritoneum approximately 1 cm below the uterovesical fold, and providing upward traction. The peritoneum is cauterized and incised perpendicular to the uterus opening the vesicovaginal space. The bladder is gently dissected and displaced downwards. The area for placement of the mesh is triangular in shape with the lower apex close to the bladder neck. The dissection is continued on the midline, close to the bladder neck to create a sufficiently large space for the attachment of the mesh anteriorly.

Dissection of the broad ligament

Dissection of the broad ligament is done at the level of the uterine isthmus, avoiding the uterine pedicles (Fig. 22.1). The uterus is slightly anteverted and displaced laterally to assist dissection of the contralateral broad ligament. The vessels of the broad ligament are cauterized and the anterior and poste-rior layers of the broad ligament incised. Care must be taken during the opening of the posterior layer of the broad ligament to avoid injury to the intestines that may be behind it. The openings in the broad ligament are then enlarged by gentle divergent traction with two instruments.

Posterior dissection

The purpose of posterior dissection is to open up the retrouterine space. The dissection begins by locating the junction of the two uterosacral ligaments at the cervix after following the course of both ureters. The peritoneum is cauterized and dissected on the midline, 2 cm below the junction of the uterosacral ligaments. The dissection is then continued to a point 1 cm from the fourchette (Fig. 22.2). This will allow treatment of a rectocele later on. This is done by fixing a Mersilene mesh to the posterior vagina and approximating the levator muscles with no. 1 Ethibond sutures.

Preparation of the sacral promontory

The patient is now placed in a Trendelenburg position. The loops of bowel are gently pushed back before the promontory can be

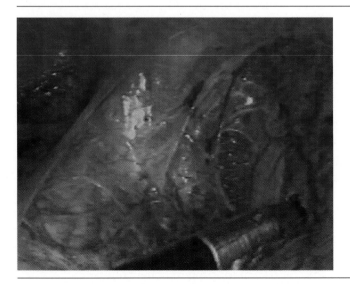

Figure 22.1 *Opening in broad ligament.*

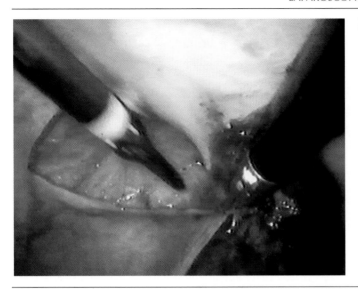

Figure 22.2 *Posterior dissection.*

safely approached. Visualization can be further improved by introducing a straight needle in the left lateral abdominal wall and knotting the suture on the skin. After identifying the right ureter and the lower border of the left common iliac vein, the posterior parietal peritoneum is incised vertically, starting from the promontory all the way to the peritoneal incision at the retrouterine space. The required fixation point is at the level of L5–S1 or the upper border of S1. The anterior longitudinal ligament is exposed. The medial sacral artery and vein are coagulated if they interfere with suturing or cannot be displaced laterally.

Fixation of the mesh in the vesicovaginal space

The Mersilene mesh is introduced through the 10-mm trocar. We prefer Mersilene mesh because of its strength and its elastic properties along the longitudinal axis. The mesh is cut in the shape of a "V", with the angle of the "V" spread out over the vesicovaginal space and the two arms of the "V" brought through the openings in the broad ligament. The length of the mesh is estimated by pushing the uterus towards L5–S1. Problems may arise if the mesh is cut too short (risk of cutting through).

The mesh is sutured to the anterior vaginal wall with a non-absorbable Ethibond 0 using a 24-mm curved needle. Extracorporeal knotting is used and six to eight interrupted sutures are required (Fig. 22.3).

The two straps of the mesh are then passed through the openings in the broad ligament and tied posteriorly at the level of the uterine isthmus (Fig. 22.4).

Anterior reperitonealization

Anterior repair of the peritoneum must be meticulous and is performed in two parts: the anterior plane for the vesicouterine peritoneum and the posterior plane for the peritoneum over the uterosacral ligaments. Continuous or interrupted suturing using Vicryl 0 and a curved needle is usually sufficient.

Posterior reperitonealization

This step is carried out to close the midline peritoneal incision between the posterior cul de sac and the promontory. Similar sutures and suturing techniques are used. Posterior reperitonealization will allow the mesh to remain in a subperitoneal position avoiding entrapment of bowel loops by an exposed mesh (Fig. 22.5). It is important to perform posterior reperitonealization before fixation of the mesh to the promontory.

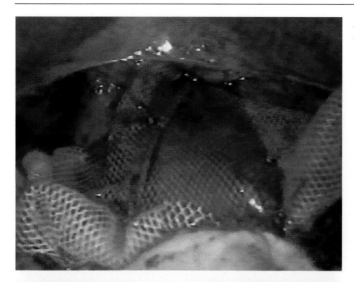

***Figure* 22.3** *Fixation of mesh in vesicovaginal space.*

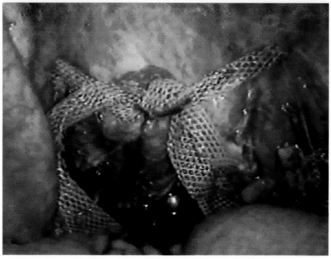

***Figure* 22.4** *Tying of mesh over posterior surface of uterus.*

Promontofixation

Promontofixation is accomplished by attaching the two mesh straps to the longitudinal vertebral ligament at the level of the promontory with two no.1 Ethibond sutures. The needle should be passed superficially over the ligament to avoid perforation of the vertebral disc and the risk of subsequent spondylitis (Fig. 22.6). After each suture is placed, traction is applied to test its strength (Fig. 22.7). For optimal results, the right amount of tension must be applied to the mesh during promontofixation and this depends on the surgeon's experience.

Burch colposuspension

Laparoscopic Burch colposuspension is often performed in conjunction with promontofixation. This procedure may benefit asymptomatic patients and those with concomitant stress incontinence. This is because excessive traction on the mesh during the promontofixation can impair the vesicourethral angle leading to postoperative stress incontinence. The authors use an intraperitoneal approach of laparoscopic Burch colposuspension. The technique is similar to that described in Chapter 20.

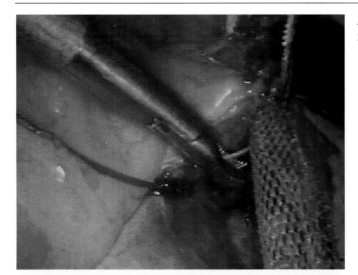

Figure 22.5 *Posterior reperitonealization.*

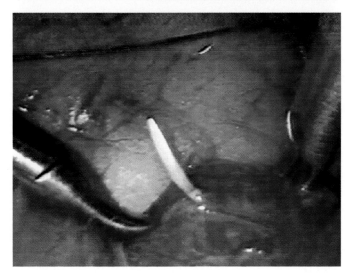

Figure 22.6 *Promontofixation.*

COMPLICATIONS

Various complications may be associated with laparoscopic promontofixation.

Complications during dissection

The two common complications that may arise during dissection of the vesicovaginal space are bleeding and bladder injury. This is often due to dissection in the wrong plane. The presence of endometriosis or previous caesaraen section may also increase the risk of bladder injury.

Bleeding of adnexal or uterine vessels is a common problem during the dissection of the broad ligament. Bowel injury is rare, but it can occur during the opening of the posterior leaf of the broad ligament.

Dissection of the rectovaginal space may lead to rectal injury. This could be avoided by dissecting as close to the vagina as possible.

Dissection to prepare the sacral promontory for fixation carries risks of injury to the bowel, the ureter (usually right) and the median sacral vessels. Visualization can be improved by a deep Trendelenburg position

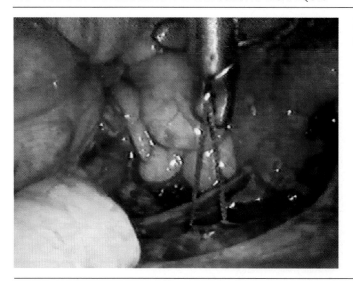

Figure 22.7 *Traction of promontory to assess strength.*

and transparietal fixation of the mesosigmoid. Injury to the medial sacral vessels can be avoided by placing the needle on the promontory not too close to the midline. Disc complications and spondylitis are also known complications of promontofixation.

Complications during mesh fixation

Loose application of the mesh can occur and this will compromise the efficacy of the procedure. On the other hand, excessive tension applied to the mesh during promontofixation may lead to urinary retention. This is due to excessive elevation of the bladder neck. Stress incontinence can also occur because of overcorrection of the prolapse leading to impairment of the urethrovesical angle.

Infection may occasionally occur. This can be reduced by avoiding entry into the vagina during laparoscopic suturing.

CONCLUSIONS

Laparoscopic promontofixation is a useful technique for the treatment of uterine pro-

lapse. It allows correction of uterine prolapse, stress incontinence, cystocele and rectocele. The technique offers all the advantages of the laparoscopic approach including shorter hospitalization, faster recovery and a rapid return to normal activity.

SUGGESTED READING

Huguier J, Scali P: La suspension posterieure de l'axe genital au disque lombo-sacra dans le traitement de certains prolapsus. *Presse Med* 1958 **66**: 781–784.

Nezhat CH, Nezhat F, Nezhat C: Laparoscopy sacral colpopexy for vaginal vault prolapse. *Obstet Gynecol* 1994 **84**: 885–888.

Scali P, Blondon J, Bethoux A *et al.*: Operations of support suspension by upper route in the treatment of vaginal prolapse. *J Gynecol Obstet Biol Reprod (Paris)* 1974 **3**: 365–378.

Timmons MC, Addison WA, Addison SB *et al.*: Abdominal sacral colpopexy in 163 women with posthysterectomy vaginal vault prolapse and enterocele. *J Reprod Med* 1992 **37**: 323–327.

Wattiez A, Boughizane S, Alexandre F *et al.*: Laparoscopic procedures for stress incontinence and prolapse. *Curr Opin Obstet Gynecol* 1995 **7**: 317–321.

23

LAPAROSCOPIC EXCISION OF RUDIMENTARY UTERINE HORN

Charles Chapron, Hervé Foulot and Jean-Bernard Dubuisson

Unicornuate uterus is the consequence of complete atresia of one of the two Mullerian ducts. They are grouped into various types according to the American Fertility Society Classification (AFS,1988):

- unicornuate uterus with a rudimentary horn with a cavity. In most cases there is no communication between the two cavities (Fig. 23.1);

- unicornuate uterus with a rudimentary horn with no cavity.

The rudimentary horn may be separated from the unicornuate uterus by fibrous tissue or adherent to it. Pregnancy can occur in the rudimentary horn with functioning endometrium, but it may lead to a uterine rupture as early as in the first trimester. A rudimentary horn that does not

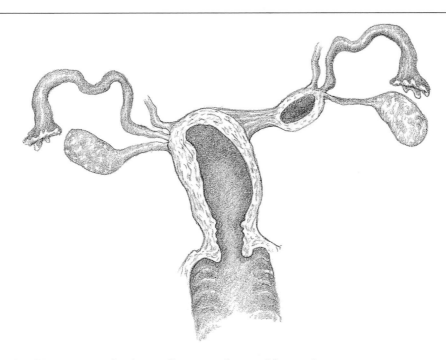

Figure 23.1 *Non-communicating rudimentary horn with a cavity.*

communicate with the unicornuate uterus results in retrograde menstruation with a risk of endometriosis.

DIAGNOSIS

The most frequent symptom is primary dysmenorrhoea, sometimes associated with dyspareunia. If the diagnosis is delayed, acute abdominal pain due to uterine rupture and haemoperitoneum can be encountered. Clinical examination may reveal an adnexal mass that corresponds to a rudimentary horn, or more commonly to an associated endometrioma.

The most useful test is ultrasonography. In order to diagnose a rudimentary horn with a cavity, ultrasonography is done in the second half of the cycle when the endometrium is more echogenic and easy to see. If there is no cavity the diagnosis is more difficult and the rudimentary horn may be confused with a subserous pedunculated myoma. An associated ovarian endometrioma can also be detected. Because of possible kidney malformation, ultrasound examination of the kidneys is indicated. An abdominopelvic scan or magnetic resonance imaging is usually unnecessary. Because of the risks of uterine horn rupture, a rudimentary horn must be excised.

PROCEDURE

1. At laparoscopy, the diagnosis should first be confirmed by the findings of a unicornuate uterus on one side, and a rudimentary horn on the opposite side. The horn may be separate from the uterus or closely attached to it. The pelvic cavity must be thoroughly inspected for endometriosis.
2. Three 5-mm suprapubic ports are recommended. In order to prevent the occurrence of tubal ectopic pregnancy, a concomitant salpingectomy should be done. This is started from the fimbrial end. The tubal ampulla is grasped using forceps placed in the ipsilateral trocar and the mesosalpinx is cauterized using bipolar coagulation. On coming close to the rudimentary horn, the tube is grasped using forceps via the opposite trocar allowing traction on the horn upwards and inwards. The round ligament is coagulated and cut. Similar to a regular hysterectomy, the peritoneum in front of the horn is opened using scissors and the bladder is pushed downwards. Haemostasis of the vessels located beneath the rudimentary horn is achieved using bipolar coagulation.
3. The rudimentary horn is now attached solely to the unicornuate uterus. Separation is easy when there is simply a strip of fibrous tissue between the rudimentary horn and the unicornuate uterus. The fibrous band is electrocoagulated and then cut. The procedure is more difficult when the horn is closely attached to the uterus. Here, separation of the rudimentary horn can be done using a monopolar hook at the point where they join. Further haemostasis is done using bipolar coagulation.
4. In the presence of endometriosis with extensive and thick adhesions, the operation must be started with lysis of these adhesions. The retroperitoneal space outside the infundibulopelvic ligament is opened, the ureter is identified and the space is further opened outside the tube. The ureter may be pushed outwards before performing salpingectomy and excision of the rudimentary horn. If there is an associated ovarian endometrioma, a laparoscopic cystectomy is done.
5. The rudimentary horn is extracted either through the 10-mm infraumbilical trocar, or in a laparoscopic pouch introduced via a 10-mm suprapubic trocar. The operation completes with careful haemostasis and liberal irrigation of the peritoneal cavity. Because patients with this condition are usually young, attention must be given to prevent adhesion formation that could adversely affect their subsequent fertility.

POTENTIAL COMPLICATIONS AND THEIR PREVENTION

In addition to complications that can occur with any laparoscopic procedure, in the presence of severe endometriosis, the ureter could be injured. Accordingly, the course of the ureter should be followed by first opening the retroperitoneal space outside the infundibulopelvic ligament. The ureter is identified and followed caudally. This is done before performing salpingectomy and excision of the rudimentary horn.

SUGGESTED READING

American Fertility Society: The American Fertility Society classifications of the adnexal adhesions, distal tubal occlusion, tubal occlusion secondary to tubal ligation, tubal pregnancy, mullerian anomalies and intra-uterine adhesions. *Fertil Steril* 1988 **49**: 944–955.

Canis M, Wattiez A, Pouly JL, Mage G, Manhes H, Bruhat MA: Laparoscopic management of unicornuate rudimentary horn and unilateral extensive endometriosis: case report. *Hum Reprod* 1990 **5**: 819–820.

Falcone T, Gidwani G, Paraiso M, Beverly C, Goldberg J: Anatomical variation in the rudimentary horns of a unicornuate uterus: implications for laparoscopic surgery. *Hum Reprod* 1997 **12**: 263–265.

Morice P, Chapron C, Garnier P, Dubuisson JB: Laparoscopic surgical ablation of a rudimentary uterine horn. *Gynaecol Endosc* 1995 **4**: 223–225.

24

LAPAROSCOPICALLY ASSISTED NEOVAGINOPLASTY

Yung Kuei Soong

Congenital absence of the vagina is a rare condition. It is estimated to be found in one of 4000–5000 female births. It may be associated with a hypoplastic uterus and rudimentary fallopian tubes. The possible aetiologies of this condition are defect in the fusion of Müllerian ducts to the urogenital sinus, Mayer–Rokitansky–Kuster–Hauser (MRKH) syndrome, and complete androgen insensitivity syndrome. There are many operative options available for the creation of a neovagina. Free skin graft or the McIndoe method, intestinal vaginoplasty, sigmoid vaginostomy, amnion graft, pedunculated skin graft, pelvic peritoneum graft and preserved human duramater grafts have all been applied to the wall of a dissected tunnel in the vesicorectal space. However, these techniques have some disadvantages. Here, a technique of laparoscopically assisted creation of a neovagina using pelvic peritoneum is described.

PROCEDURE

1. Under general anaesthesia and Trendelenburg position, the intra-abdominal organs are thoroughly inspected. Two suprapubic 5-mm trocars are inserted into the abdominal cavity at the level of anterior superior iliac spines and lateral to the epigastric blood vessels.
2. Relaxing peritoneal incisions are made lateral to the infundibulopelvic ligament on each side and over the bladder (Fig. 24.1). This is to facilitate pulling down of the loosest, most pendulous, deep cul-de-sac peritoneum to the vaginal introitus.
3. Dissection of the pelvic peritoneum over the pouch of Douglas is delicately performed to make a continuation with the bilateral pelvic incisions.

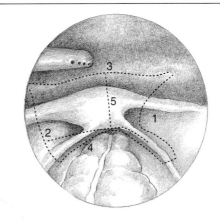

Figure 24.1 *Five steps for relaxing pelvic peritoneum by laparoscopy. Steps 1 and 2: peritoneal incisional line lateral to right and left infundibulopelvic ligaments. Step 3: incisional line over the bladder peritoneal reflection. Step 4: dissection of the pelvic peritoneum over the pouch of Douglas to make a continuation with the bilateral pelvic incisions. Step 5: excision of the uterine remnant.*

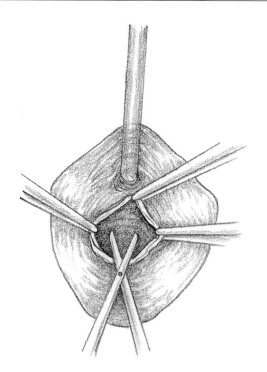

Figure 24.2

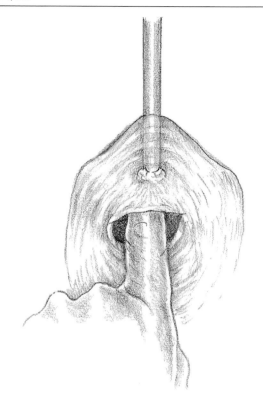

Figure 24.3

Figures 24.2 and 24.3 *A vaginal opening is created by dissection of the new vaginal canal in the plane between the bladder and rectum via a vaginal approach by the surgeons index finger in the vagina.*

4. Complete excision of the uterine remnants through the central incisional line is performed after the peritoneum is relaxed. The hypoplastic uterus is removed before excision of the peritoneum.
5. A vaginal opening is created by blunt dissection of the new vaginal canal in the plane between the bladder and rectum via a vaginal approach by the surgeon's index finger in the vagina (Figs 24.2 and 24.3). This is assisted with scissors via laparoscopy. Complete haemostasis is mandatory when creating this space.
6. After the peritoneum is reached, a Kelly clamp is inserted transvaginally to grasp and pull down the previously relaxed peritoneum, and the tip of the peritoneum is then anchored with 0-Vicryl sutures to the edge of the neovaginal orifice on each side (Fig. 24.4).
7. A temporary vaginal stent made of a wick of gauze around a 20-ml syringe or a plastic mould is inserted into the previously prepared vaginal space.
8. The abdominal peritoneal incision is closed by 2-0-Vicryl sutures or using an endoscopic stapler.
9. One week later the stent is removed and a neovagina is created.

Postoperatively, the patient is taught to apply a glass dilator to maintain the length and width of the neovagina. Dilatation is done four times a day for 1 h and during the sleep period for a minimum of 3 months. Two different dilators are used, a 11.5-cm length dilator for creating depth and a 3.0-cm dilator for maintaining the width of the neovagina.

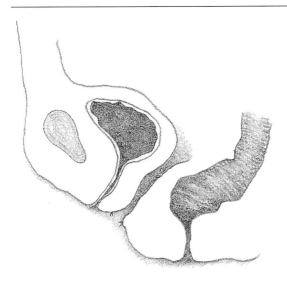

Figure 24.4 *After the peritoneum is reached, a Kelly clamp is inserted transvaginally to grasp and pull down the previously relaxed peritoneum, and the tip of the peritoneum is anchored with 0-Vicryl sutures to the edge of the neovaginal orifice on each side.*

ALTERNATIVE TECHNIQUES

Other techniques of laparoscopically assisted neovaginoplasty have also been reported. These include a technique described by Vecchietti. The instrumentation consists of a traction device, suture ligature carriers and an acrylic shaped olive measuring 2.2 × 1.9 cm. The procedure is done by first incising the peritoneum between the bladder and the rectum. This is followed by dissection between these two organs. A straight ligature carrier is then passed transabdominally through the space between the rectum and the bladder, piercing the perineum between the labia. The acrylic olive is threaded into a suture and is pulled to the peritoneum by the suture that is attached to a traction device on the abdominal wall. Constant and increasing traction of the acrylic olive by the traction device produces invagination of the space between the bladder and the rectum creating a neovagina. By using this gradual traction, a neovagina is created in 7–9 days. However, in my opinion, this technique is complicated and time consuming. Furthermore, it needs special instrumentation.

POSSIBLE COMPLICATIONS AND THEIR PREVENTION

Bleeding can occur during the dissection of the space between the rectum and the vagina. Injury to the bladder or the rectum may also occur. Gentle dissection and meticulous haemostasis are mandatory.

SUGGESTED READING

Veronikis DH, McLure GB, Nichols DH: The Vecchietti operation for constructing a neo-vagina: indications, instrumentation, and techniques. *Obstet Gynecol* 1997 **90**: 301–304.

25

OFFICE LAPAROSCOPY

Joseph Feste

Since Jacobaeus performed the first laparoscopy in 1910, surgeons have made great strides in utilizing this valuable tool. Unfortunately, the expense of performing even diagnostic laparoscopy has become prohibitive. With the high cost of medical care, measures must be taken to decrease this monumental problem. For years, laparoscopy has been performed under local anaesthesia with minimal reported complications. In most of the reported cases, a 10-mm trocar was used, especially for tubal sterilization. With this vast experience, a method of simpler laparoscopy has been proposed.

The first few procedures were performed with a prototype 1.8-mm outer diameter microlaparoscope developed by Medical Dynamics Inc. (Englewood, Colorado). A more advanced catheter called "Pixie" microendoscope was provided by Origin Medsystems, Inc. (Menlo Park, CA.) (Fig. 25.1) The depth of field with the Origin Pixie microendoscope is 150 mm compared to approximately 25 mm with the Medical Dynamics microlaparoscope. The greater depth of field is similar to the field of vision of a diagnostic laparoscope 5–10 mm in outer diameter. The microendoscope was attached to a video camera with a light source and monitor. A third microendoscopic device, the "MicroLap Gold" (Imagyn Medical, New Jersey) (Fig. 25.2), has a depth of field of 100 mm, an external diameter of

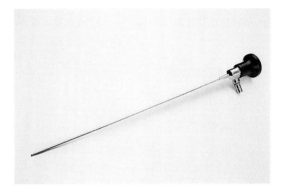

Figure 25.1 A 1.98-mm microlaparoscope (Origin).

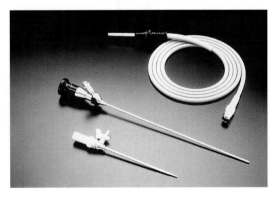

Figure 25.2 A 3-mm microlaparoscope (Micro-Lap Gold, Imagyn).

1.98 mm, 50,000 pixels of light and resolution similar to a 5 mm diagnostic laparoscope. The eyepiece of this microlaparoscope can be attached to any video camera system.

Olympus has manufactured a fourth micro-endoscope. This instrument has an outer diameter of 3 mm and a custom trocar made by Ethicon.

Microlaparoscopy can be done under local anaesthesia, in an office setting, is a less technical procedure, and is significantly less expensive. It is convenient for the surgeon by saving time out of office and travelling time. It will save time waiting in the operative suite at hospital for another physician to finish. It is less inconvenient for the patient; it facilitates several processes including the admissions process, anaesthesia standby and laboratory visit. Patient acceptance will require education as to the benefits of the procedure and the ease with which it can be done.

INDICATIONS

Second-look laparoscopy for adhesion assessment

In patients who have had stage IV endometriosis or adhesive disease treated by laparoscopy or by laparotomy, the incidence of postoperative adhesions is high (up to 90%). Yet, 34% of patients with minimal adhesions would have to undergo an unnecessary laparoscopy if one were to laparoscope all these patients. By using a microlaparoscope in the office, only patients who need adhesiolysis would be required to undergo another surgery.

In order to facilitate the microlaparoscopy, a Tenckhoff catheter is placed in the umbilicus, cutting the inside portion of the catheter about 2 inches (5 cm) from the inside peritoneum at the time of the initial surgical procedure. The catheter is taped to the abdomen with a waterproof tape. The patient returns to the office or hospital treatment room for an "office laparoscopy". Under local anaesthesia, a 1.98-mm microlaparoscope is inserted through the Tenckhoff catheter as a trocar, and the abdominal cavity is inspected. If the patient is found to have no or minimal adhesions, no further action is taken. Otherwise, the adhesions can be separated with a laparoscopic probe. At one-week after the intial surgery, the adhesions are soft and can be separated easily (Fig. 25.3). Spraying local anaesthesia on the area will reduce the pain. Extensive and dense adhesions require lysis under general anaesthesia. In order to determine the likelihood of requiring general anaesthesia, the decision is made at the time of the initial surgery. If the initial operation is associated with cohesive or vascular adhesions involving the adnexa, these patients should be scheduled in the operating room but under local (possibly general) anaesthesia. Accord-

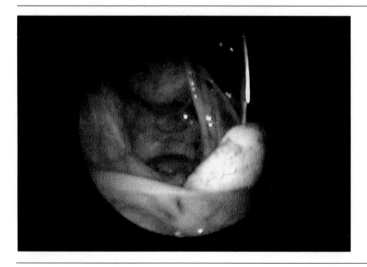

Figure 25.3 Microlaparoscopic view of periadnexal adhesion.

ingly, the patient will benefit from the lower cost of local microlaparoscopy but have the option to have the treatment completed should more extensive adhesions be found.

Suspected endometriosis and chronic pelvic pain with minimal or no physical findings (pain mapping)

By using office laparoscopy, endometriosis can be classified (Fig. 25.4) and the aetiology of pelvic pain can be evaluated. In patients with no obvious physical findings for over three months and not relieved by standard medical therapy, evaluation with the micro-laparoscope would be beneficial. However, whether the findings are the cause of the pain remain uncertain. This could be evaluated by inserting a secondary 3-mm trocar in the midline. A 2-mm grasper is used to gently pull the adhesion or peritoneum over the endometriotic implant and ask the patient if the pain has been duplicated (Fig. 25.5). Accordingly, it is important that the patient is not overly sedated. Local anaesthesia and Versed are appropriate for this purpose.

Tubal sterilization

Tubal sterilization has been performed under local anaesthesia for many years. A smaller endoscope would decrease the

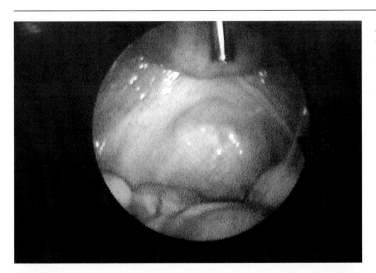

Figure 25.4 Microlaparoscopic view of endometriosis on the left uterosacral ligament.

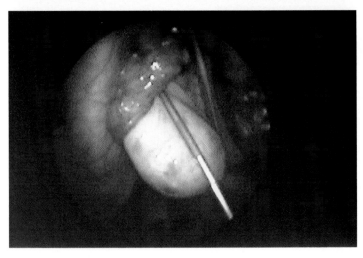

Figure 25.5 Pelvic mapping for chronic pelvic pain. The probe is touching the right ovary and fallopian tube.

likelihood of complications as well as provide more than adequate vision for tubal coagulation or other methods of sterilization. The recovery time is shorter and the amount of pain associated with the procedure is minimal. The obvious decrease in cost over the conventional laparoscopy makes this procedure attractive to patients with no insurance coverage and to the insurance company as well.

The key to successful tubal sterilization by microlaparoscopy is to utilize a significant amount of local anaesthesia, within 10% of the maximum dose allowed. Spraying the tubes with local anaesthesia also decreases the amount of discomfort. The procedure can be performed with a 2 or 3-mm trocar within the umbilicus and a 5-mm "Step" trocar that can be radially dilated from 5 to 8 mm for the purpose of applying a Filshie clip. For those patients with low pain threshold, conscious sedation can be given.

Infertility

Frequently, infertility is often not covered by insurance and office laparoscopy can be cost-effective.

The above are the most commonly utilized four procedures done under local or conscious sedation. The availability of stand-by anaesthesia in the operating room allows conversion to general anaesthestic laparoscopy if needed. The surgeon should identify which patients should be treated in an alternate site versus in the operating room with stand-by anaesthesia. Other indications for microlaparoscopy in the operating room include evaluation of abdominal pain (appendicitis versus salpingitis), possible ruptured ovarian cyst, leaking ectopic pregnancy with or without methotrexate therapy and adnexal torsion. Other procedures that might utilize the microlaparoscope in an office setting would be postoperative evaluation of neosalpingostomy before gamete or zygote intrafallopian transfer.

EQUIPMENT

The procedure is performed in an out-patient setting either in the hospital minor procedure room, operating room or office treatment room. The equipment needed to perform the procedure is as follows (Fig. 25.6):

1. Microlaparoscope system including a microlaparoscope, light cord, video camera, light source and monitor;
2. Pulse oximeter and blood pressure cuff;
3. Table capable of Trendelenburg;
4. Microlaparoscope, Veress needle with trocar;

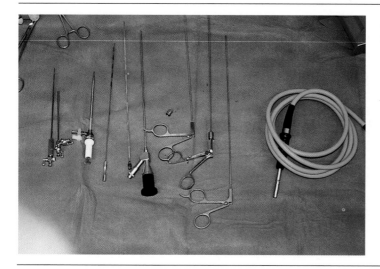

Figure 25.6 Equipment used in microlaparoscopy.

5. CO$_2$ insufflator (nitrous oxide is preferred except for sterilization);
6. Sterile drapes and Band-Aids;
7. Heparin-lock (18–22 gauge) for injection of i.v. analgesics or sedatives;
8. Betadine prep tray;
9. Intrauterine cannula;
10. Speculum;
11. Local anaesthesia (1–2% nesacaine);
12. 2-mm and 5-mm trocars for ancillary instruments (Step Trocar);
13. Bipolar forceps for sterilization;
14. Microlaparoscopic instruments.

Anaesthesia

The selection of the proper local anaesthetic depends on the procedure to be performed. Since microlaparoscopy is generally a short procedure, one needs to use a drug that is fast acting, mild to moderate potency, and has a wide margin of safety. Nesacaine appears to be the best choice. However, if the procedure is potentially longer than usual, one might select marcaine, which has a much longer lasting effect. Unfortunately, the maximal dose is only up to 200 mg for the entire procedure. Injecting three or four puncture sites plus adding local anaesthesia within the pelvic cavity may quickly use up the allotted amount of drug. In all cases except for evaluation of pelvic pain one can use more ancillary medication to promote pain relief and use less local anaesthetic.

It is important to monitor the maximum amount of drug used. Injections of these anaesthetic drugs have to be properly monitored with no intravenous injection allowed. Only a small amount of drug given intravenously can be catastrophic. A "crash cart" should always be available in the vicinity of the minor procedure room.

PROCEDURE

1. The patient is asked to empty her bladder then she is positioned in as deep Trendelenburg as she can tolerate. A blood pressure cuff and pulse oximeter is attached to the patient's arm and finger. A 21-gauge heplock is inserted into her arm for intravenous medication. Two mg of Versed is given 15 minutes before the procedure and 0.4 mg of Robinol to prevent a vagal reaction. In most cases, additional Versed 2–6 mg i.v. titrated prior to making the incision for insertion of the Veress needle is given. Additional Valium, Fentanil or Versed can be administered as needed.
2. A paracervical block is performed and an intrauterine cannula is inserted. A generous amount of local anaesthesia is injected through all layers of the abdominal wall (Fig. 25.7). A small incision is made in the skin and the Veress needle within the microtrocar sheath is introduced into the

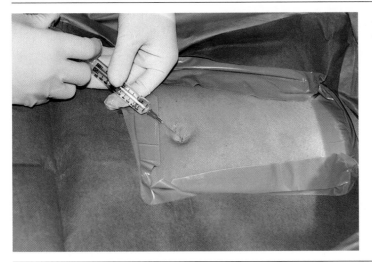

Figure 25.7 *Injection of local anaesthesia in the umbilical area.*

abdominal cavity at a 45° angle with the uterus being held down by an intrauterine cannula (Fig. 25.8). The Veress needle is removed from the plastic sheath and a gas extension tube is connected to the CO_2 insufflator. Approximately 500–600 ml of CO_2 or nitrous oxide is instilled into the peritoneal cavity. Nitrous oxide is less irritating to the peritoneal surfaces and is absorbed rapidly. However, many operating rooms have restrictions for using nitrous oxide.

3. Another 2-mm trocar or 5-mm "Step Trocar" (InnerDyne, Sunnyvale, CA) can be inserted suprapubically (Fig. 25.9) to aspirate fluid, to manipulate the viscera, to perform sterilization, to liberate adhesions or to take cultures or biopsies. This port can also be used to insert a 100-μm laser fibre or a bipolar cautery to liberate adhesions or to vaporize endometriotic implants. Following the procedure, the gas is removed before taking the patient out of Trendelenburg position and steristrips are placed over the incision. The patient is allowed to sit up and should be observed for 30–45 min before discharge.

CONTRAINDICATIONS

Contraindications for the use of the microlaparoscope are similar to those of laparo-

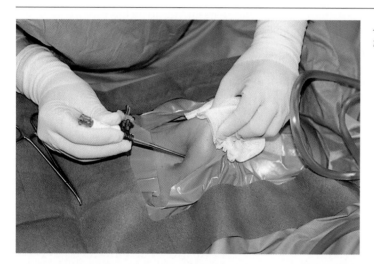

Figure 25.8 Insertion of a microtrocar.

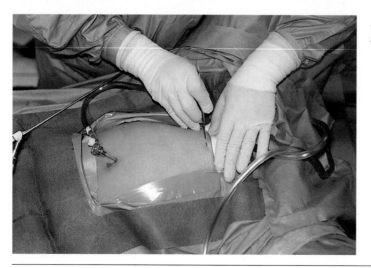

Figure 25.9 Another incision for a secondary trocar suprapubically.

scopy in general. Patients with a history of multiple operations would be a relative contraindication for an office laparoscopy.

SUGGESTED READING

Childers MD, Hatch KD, Surwit MD: Office laparoscopy and biopsy for evaluation of patients with intraperitoneal carcinomatosis using a new microlaparoscope. *Gynecol Oncol* 1992 **47**: 337–342.

Feste JR: The use of optical catheters for diagnostic office laparoscopy. *J Reprod* 1996 309–312.

Fishburne JI: Office laparoscopic sterilization with local anaesthesia. *J Reprod Med* 1977 **18**: 233–234.

Jansen RS: Early laparoscopy after pelvic operations to prevent adhesions: safety and efficacy. *Fertil Steril* 1988 **49**: 26–31.

Penfield AJ: Laparoscopic sterilization under local anaesthesia *J Reprod Med* 1974 **12**: 251.

Steege JF, Stout AL, Somkuti SG: Chronic pelvic pain in women: toward an integrative model. *Obstet Gynecol Surg* 1993 **48**: 95–110.

26

LAPAROSCOPY IN PREGNANCY

Salli I. Tazuke, Farr R. Nezhat, Ceana H. Nezhat, Daniel S. Seidman, Maurizio Rosati and Camran R. Nezhat

Operative laparoscopy was revolutionized with the incorporation of a camera and video equipment in the mid 1980s. As surgeons gained more experience in operative laparoscopy, the procedure was expanded to the pregnant population. However, treatment of pregnant patients requires consideration of the well-being of both the mother and the fetus, and the associated abdominal pathologies. Surgery during pregnancy may be associated with increased fetal morbidity and mortality. The displacement of intraabdominal organs by the gravid uterus also makes the diagnosis of certain pathology more difficult (Figs 26.1 and 26.2). Accordingly, many clinicians have reserved surgical intervention until absolutely necessary. Such a tendency to delay surgical intervention is often associated with increased morbidity of both the mother and the fetus. Thus, the management of possible surgical abdominal pathology in pregnant patients renders significant clinical challenge to the clinician.

Literature on successful laparoscopic intervention during pregnancy is largely limited to case reports. One case-control study comparing the outcome of laparoscopic appendectomy and cholecystectomy with that of laparotomy during the first two trimesters demonstrated that laparoscopic surgery significantly decreased hospitalization and the amount of narcotic use. Also, the bowel function returned rapidly, and no

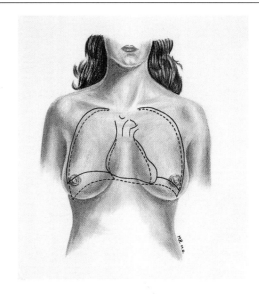

Figure 26.1 *Displacement of the diaphragm, the lung and the heart during pregnancy. ——, pregnant; – – –, non-pregnant.*

differences were noted in the gestational age at delivery, Apgar scores, birth weights, or other complications. The composite of these experiences affirms that laparoscopic surgery is indeed feasible during pregnancy and suggests that pregnant patients may also benefit from the less-invasive surgical approach. However, questions remain as to whether laparoscopic surgery is as safe as laparotomy for the fetus and expectant

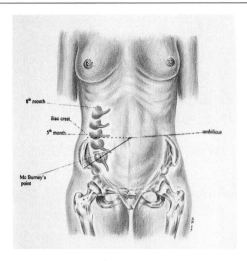

Figure 26.2 *Position of appendix vermiformis with advancing age of gestation.*

mother and caution is warranted until further evidence accumulates.

LAPAROSCOPIC PROCEDURES IN PREGNANCY

Diagnostic laparoscopy

For many years, gynecologic surgeons performed diagnostic laparoscopies in pregnant women in the first trimester to rule out ectopic pregnancy. Most resulted in normal intrauterine pregnancies, and exposure to laparoscopy *per se* did not appear to have adverse effects on the pregnancy.

Appendectomy

Appendicitis is the most common indication for non-obstetric abdominal surgery during pregnancy. It occurs in about 0.5–1 per 1000 pregnancies. Appendicitis in pregnancy poses diagnostic and management challenges due to the displacement of the appendix by the gravid uterus (Fig. 26.2). Hampered by the lack of sensitive and specific non-invasive tests during pregnancy, a false positive preoperative diagnosis up to one-third of the time is accepted as the norm. The fear of surgical intervention in a preg-

nant woman, compounded by the diagnostic difficulty frequently lead to delay in surgical intervention until absolutely necessary. Operation in advanced stage of appendicitis is associated with higher morbidity. Furthermore, perforation of the appendix is followed by a dramatic increase in fetal mortality.

Cholecystectomy

For cholecystectomy, the literature is more abundant and supportive of the laparoscopic approach. Cholecystitis occurs in 1:600 to 1:10,000 pregnancies and is the second most common indication for non-obstetric surgical intervention in pregnancy. Laparoscopic cholecystectomy has been done even during the third trimester. This is due to the unchanged location of the gall bladder in the right upper quadrant. However, the risk of damage to the uterus during the procedure is increased, and wide application of laparoscopic cholecystectomy during the third trimester may not be warranted.

Adnexal Surgery

A common indication for surgical intervention during pregnancy is persistent adnexal mass. The majority of these are cysts that will spontaneously regress by 15–16 weeks gestation. Persistence beyond 15–16 weeks gestation and size greater than 5–6 cm are associated with increasing risk of torsion, rupture, dystocia and malignancy, justifying surgical diagnosis and removal of the mass in question.

Heterotopic pregnancy

From 1990 to 1996, there were seven cases of laparoscopic removal of heterotopic pregnancies published in the literature. They were at gestational age between 6 and 10 weeks, and involved either salpingectomy or cornual resection of an interstitial pregnancy. All the associated *in utero* pregnancies progressed normally into the third trimester. Thus, pelvic operative laparoscopy appears to be not only feasible but safe during pregnancy in the first trimester.

PROCEDURE

1. Because of the enlarged uterus, extra care must be taken with trocar insertion. An open laparoscopic approach may be taken, or alternatively, the primary and secondary trocar insertion sites can be modified to either supraumbilical or sub-xiphoid midline, or left upper quadrant. The primary insertion site is best determined after palpating the uterine fundus, and the ancillary trocars are placed under direct visualization (Fig. 26.3). The use of Veress needle has resulted in inadvertent uterine insufflation and is not recommended during pregnancy.

2. In the presence of a pregnancy or a possible pregnancy, no instrument should be applied to the cervix or inserted into the uterine cavity.

3. Impaired venous return via compression of the inferior vena cava by the enlarged uterus is of particular concern in the second half of pregnancy. The uterine compression of the vena cava can be reduced by slight lateral positioning of the mother, as is commonly done during Caesarean section.

4. The risk of hypercarbia and acidosis should be minimized by maintaining the intra-abdominal pressure to less than 12 mmHg and short operative time.

5. The effect of carbon dioxide pneumo-peritoneum on fetal well-being remains unknown. Gasless laparoscopy has been advocated, but its efficacy remains unclear. Similarly, the safety of pneumo-peritoneum using nitrous oxide versus carbon dioxide (CO_2) gas is still unknown.

POTENTIAL COMPLICATIONS AND THEIR PREVENTION

1. Injury to the uterus and CO_2 embolism secondary to insufflation into the uterine cavity. This can be avoided by open laparoscopy or modifying the site of trocar insertion. The trocar must be directed well away from the uterus at the time of insertion.

2. Maternal hypercarbia due to upward displacement of diaphragm, decreased venous return due to the enlarged

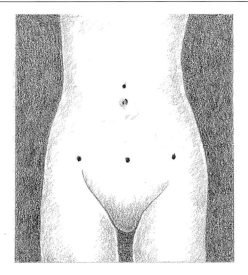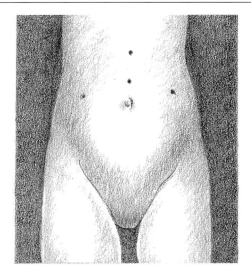

Figure 26.3 Trocar sites for operative laparoscopy in early pregnancy (left) and in second trimester of pregnancy (right).

uterus and Trendelenberg position and possible fetal hypoxia. Both the surgeon and the anaesthetist should pay particular attention to proper positioning of the mother. Supine recumbency should be avoided and the hip should be tilted by at least 15°. The haemodynamic and respiratory variables should be monitored closely during surgery and the length of operative time kept to a minimum.

3. Pregnancy demise. This may be more related to the underlying condition itself rather than the surgical intervention, particularly when an inflammatory or infectious process is involved.

4. Cervical and intra-abdominal manipulation both increase the risk of premature labour. The risk further increases when the underlying pathology includes an inflammatory or infectious process and fever. This is well established in cases of appendicitis, when perforation of the appendix is associated with a fourfold increase in the risk of premature labour.

5. An additional potential danger is the risk of exposure to intra-abdominal smoke generated by electrosurgery and laser, with resultant production of increased levels of noxious gases, most importantly carbon monoxide. We recently measured the levels of serum carboxyhaemoglobin in women undergoing prolonged operative laparoscopy procedures. No increase in the levels of carboxyhaemoglobin was detected, and this was attributed to rapid evacuation of intra-abdominal smoke generated during surgery.

6. The effect of pneumoperitoneum and intra-abdominal CO_2 on the fetus remains unknown. These issues must be carefully weighed and considered with laparoscopic approach.

CONCLUSIONS

Abdominal and pelvic pathology necessitating surgical intervention during pregnancy represents a clinical challenge to the obstetrician/gynecologist. The underlying pathology and the surgical intervention pose certain risks to the gravid patient and the fetus. In general, the surgical intervention can be safe particularly when there is no inflammatory process or fever, and when manipulation of uterus and cervix is avoided.

Operative laparoscopy is increasingly being utilized for various indications due to its known advantages and benefits. Pregnant patients may also benefit from the less invasive nature of the laparoscopic approach. Concerns remain, particularly regarding the effect of CO_2 pneumoperitoneum on maternal haemodynamics and associated potential for fetal asphyxia. More prospective randomized studies are needed to accurately assess the safety, efficacy, and advantages of operative laparoscopy over laparotomy and great care must be taken in the meantime.

SUGGESTED READING

Laparoscopy. In Nezhat CR, Nezhat FR, Luciano AA, Siegler AM, Metzger DA and Nezhat CH (eds) *Operative Gynecologic Laparoscopy: Principles and Techniques*. McGraw-Hill, New York, 1995, pp. 79–96.

Barron WM: Medical evaluation of the pregnant patient requiring nonobstetric surgery. *Clin Perinatol* 1985 **12**: 481–496.

Callery MP, Soper NJ: Physiology of the pneumoperitoneum. *Baillière's Clin Gastroenterol* 1993 **7**: 757–777.

Curet MJ, Allen D, Josloff RK, Pitcher DE, Curet LB, Miscall BG, Zucker KA: Laparoscopy during pregnancy. *Arch Surg* 1996 **131**: 546–551.

Nezhat FR, Tazuke S, Nezhat CH, Seidman DS, Phillips DR, Nezhat CR: Laparoscopy during pregnancy: a literature review. *J Soc Laparoendosc Surg* 1997 **1**: 17–27.

27

GASLESS LAPAROSCOPY

Yung Kuei Soong

Several authors have reported the utilization of abdominal distention systems without pneumoperitoneum in providing adequate exposure for laparoscopic operations. This approach is called gasless laparoscopy. Here, the conventional laparotomy instruments such as clamps, scissors, tenaculum and others can be used. During coagulation, the vapour escapes immediately through open trocars and a conventional suction tube can be utilized without loss of abdominal distention. In the absence of pneumoperitoneum, significant metabolic and haemodynamic changes associated with carbon dioxide gas are avoided.

In the author's opinion, it is useful especially for laparoscopic myomectomy. Laparoscopic myomectomy, especially for large leiomyoma can be troublesome and is a tedious procedure. It is associated with increased operating time and it requires a skilled laparoscopist. It is also difficult to repair the uterus in layers by laparoscopy, and hence it is harder to control the bleeding. The risks of uteroperitoneal fistula formation and uterine dehiscence are theoretically increased. Myomectomy using gasless laparoscopic approach has some advantages over the conventional laparoscopy in the surgical treatment of large leiomyoma. For infertility procedures, it appears that there is no difference in postoperative discomfort after conventional laparoscopy and gasless laparoscopy. In

fact, gasless laparoscopy increases technical difficulty.

PROCEDURE

Preoperative preparation consists of three days minimal residue diet to reduce bowel gas. Under general anaesthesia with a nasogastric tube, a gasless laparoscopy is performed using an airlift balloon retractor. The airlift balloon retraction system consists of one balloon retractor and one Laparolift arm (Origin Medsystems Inc.). It is designed to be used for retracting the abdominal wall during laparoscopic surgery (Fig. 27.1). Instead of airlift balloon, a disposable device consisting of two 10 or 15-cm blades and a handle (Laparofan, Origin Medsystems Inc) that attaches to the Laparolift can also be utilized. The Laparolift is fixed to the right side of the operating table. The procedure is performed with the patient in a Trendelenburg position.

A 2-cm skin incision is made in the base of the umbilicus and deepens through the fascia and peritoneum. A deflated airlift balloon is introduced into the incision until the entire sheathed portion enters the peritoneal cavity. Once in a correct position, the balloon is inflated by pumping the inflation-electrically powered lifting device attached to the side rail of the operating table. This Laparolift is elevated to the desired height and the suspension system is used to raise

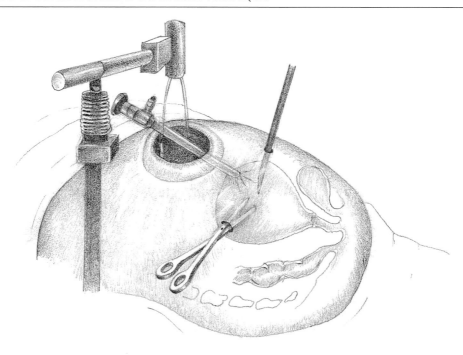

Figure 27.1 A schematic diagram of a gasless-laparoscopic myomectomy. Note conventional laparotomy instruments are used.

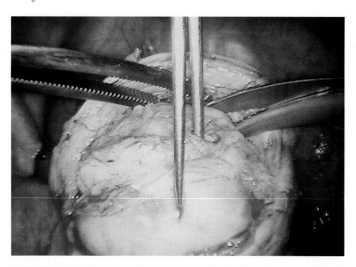

Figure 27.2 Myomectomy using gasless-laparoscopic approach. (Courtesy of Howard Topel MD.)

the abdominal wall. When fully deployed, the balloon is a 5 inch (13 cm) donut-shaped structure with a 5-cm central opening. Thereafter, the laparoscope and another instrument can be inserted simultaneously though the central ring of the airlift balloon. Two additional valveless 10-mm trocars are placed under direct vision along the mid-clavicular line, one at the right side of the

anterior superior iliac spine and another at the opposite side (Fig. 27.2). Through these incisions, conventional instruments including a long scalpel, Metzenbaum scissors and tenaculum can be used. Magnification is obtained by bringing the tip of the laparoscope closed to the tissue.

This gasless laparoscopic approach allows the use of a conventional long needle holder for suturing. Knots are tied directly by the surgeon's finger. In most cases, half-hitch knots are created extracorporeally and are guided into place with an index finger inserted through the suprapubic incision. Specimen is removed through the suprapubic incision. Usually, the incision is enlarged to 2 cm to allow delivery of the entire specimen out of the abdominal cavity. When postoperative oozing is expected, a drain is inserted through the suprapubic puncture and removed the following day. Incisions are closed in a standard fashion after the removal of retractors and trocars.

POTENTIAL COMPLICATIONS AND CONTRAINDICATIONS

The complication rate of gasless laparoscopy is considerably less than that of conventional laparoscopy. Obesity is a relative contraindication to this laparoscopic approach. In obese women, a larger incision is needed to gain access into the abdominal cavity.

SUGGESTED READING

Chang FH, Soong YK, Lee CL, Lai YM, Wang HS: Laparoscopic myomectomy of a large symptomatic leiomyoma using airlift gasless laparoscopy. *Hum Reprod* 1996 **11**: 1427–1432.

Goldberg JM, Maurer WG: A randomized comparison of gasless laparoscopy and CO_2 pneumoperitoneum. *Obstet Gynecol* 1997 **90**: 416–420.

28

LAPAROSCOPIC SALPINGOSCOPY

Riccardo Marana, Paul Caruana, Giovan Fiore Catalano, Ludovico Muzii and Salvatore Mancuso

Salpingoscopy is an endoscopic technique that allows direct evaluation of the tubal mucosa. Indications for salpingoscopy include history of salpingitis, tubal reconstructive surgery and previous tubal pregnancy. Tubal factor infertility accounts for approximately 40% of cases of female infertility. Identifiable causes of tubal infertility are postinfectious tubal damage, endometriosis-related adhesions and post-surgical adhesion formation.

Reproductive surgery is performed with the aim of allowing ovum pick-up by restoring normal anatomical relationships between the fimbriae and the ovary. However, although reproductive surgery may be successful in restoring normal anatomy, it does not restore normal function of the tubal mucosa. Pregnancy outcome following tubal reconstructive surgery for distal tubal occlusion (DTO) and adnexal adhesions is related to the extent of tubal disease and pelvic adhesions. Based on the various parameters, several classification systems have been proposed to assess the extent of tubal disease in order to predict pregnancy outcome. In 1988 the American Fertility Society (AFS) proposed a scoring system based on the extent and type of adhesions, thickness and rigidity of the tubal wall, distal ampullary diameter, and percentage of mucosal folds preserved at the neostomy site. The importance of intraoperative salpingoscopy to visualize the entire length of the ampullary mucosa as an important prognostic parameter was recognized. However, salpingoscopic findings were not included in the scoring system as salpingoscopy was done only in a few centres.

PROCEDURE

Salpingoscopy allows direct evaluation of the endosalpinx following distention of the ampullary segment of the tube using Ringer's lactate solution. It necessitates a laparoscope with a 7-mm operative channel. The instruments include a 2.8-mm rigid salpingoscope, a salpingoscope sheath with a rounded tip obturator and atraumatic tube-grasping forceps. The outer sheath is connected through an infusion set to a flask of Ringer's lactate solution placed approximately 1 m above the patient. The hydrostatic pressure of the solution at this height moderately distends the tubal wall thus allowing clear visualization of the tubal mucosa. Under direct laparoscopic vision the tube to be examined is aligned with the axis of the laparoscope. In most cases this may be achieved by manipulating the uterine corpus into the ipsilateral ovarian fossa using a Cohen's cannula after elevating the adnexa using a probe introduced through a suprapubic trocar sleeve. After these manipulations, the ovary and fallopian tube should be resting over the anterior uterine wall (Fig. 28.1). The

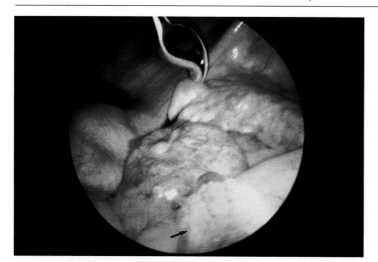

Figure 28.1a

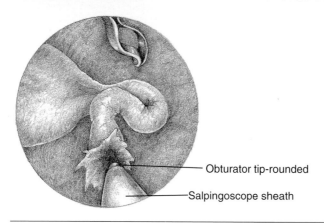

Obturator tip-rounded

Salpingoscope sheath

Figure 28.1b

Figures 28.1a and b *The tube is positioned over the anterior wall of the uterus. The salpingoscope sheath containing the rounded tip oburator is seen* (arrow).

peritoneal ostium of the tube is identified and cannulated with the outer sheath of the salpingoscope containing the rounded tip obturator. When there is distal tubal occlusion, the tube should be incised at the site of fimbrial conglutination and the tube cannulated through the site of incision (Fig. 28.2). The distal portion of the tube is then clamped around the outer sheath by means of the atraumatic tube-holding forceps introduced through the suprapubic trocar sleeve (Fig. 28.3). The obturator is withdrawn and replaced by the salpingoscope. The infusion set is opened and the salpingoscope is delicately advanced into the tube under direct vision.

COMPLICATIONS AND THEIR PREVENTION

It is unlikely that salpingoscopy is associated with complications. However, rough handling of the fimbriae can lead to fimbrial damage, bleeding and adhesion formation. Preferably the fimbriae should not be handled at all. The tube should be cannulated with the outer sheath containing the rounded tip obturator and only then clamped at the infundibular level around the outer sheath using the atraumatic tube-holding forceps.

Perforation of the tube may occur when introducing the sheath, but more likely, if the salpingoscope is advanced blindly and roughly. The technique necessitates extremely gentle handling of the tube.

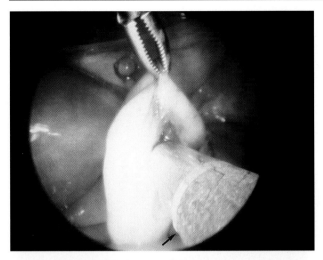

Figure 28.2 *Distal tubal occlusion: the salpingoscope sheath is seen during cannulation of the tube through the site of incision* (arrow).

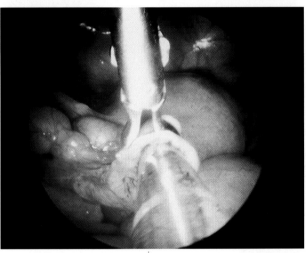

Figure 28.3 *The tube is aligned with the long axis of the laparoscope. The tube is clamped around the infundibulum using the atraumatic tube-holding forceps.*

CLASSIFICATION OF THE STATUS OF TUBAL MUCOSA

At the ampullary level four or five major folds are noted with minor folds interspersed between them. The major folds have a fine capillary network and secondary folds may be seen arising from them. The status of the tubal mucosa should be classified according to the classification proposed by Puttemans *et al.* (1987) as follows: grade I, normal mucosal folds are seen (Fig. 28.4); grade II, the major folds are separated and flattened but otherwise normal (in fact, this might be considered a grade I tube distended by increased intraluminal hydrostatic pressure); grade III, focal adhesions are seen between the mucosal folds (Figs 28.5 and 28.6); grade IV, extensive adhesions are present between the mucosal folds and/or disseminated flat areas (Fig. 28.7); grade V, there is a complete loss of the mucosal fold pattern (Fig. 28.8).

PROGNOSTIC VALUE OF SALPINGOSCOPY

In 1995, we reported on a series of 55 patients operated on either by microsurgery or by laparoscopy for tubal infertility and submitted to concomitant salpingoscopy.

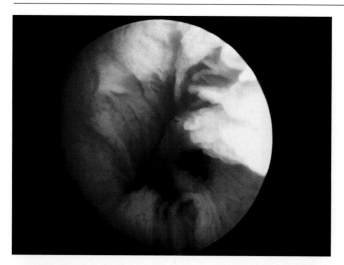

Figure 28.4 Salpingoscopic grade I: normal ampullary mucosa.

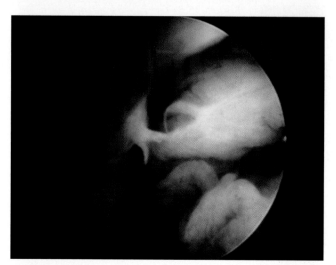

Figure 28.5 Salpingoscopic grade III: note the presence of focal adhesions.

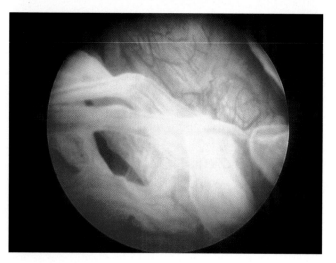

Figure 28.6 Salpingoscopic grade III: note the presence of focal adhesions.

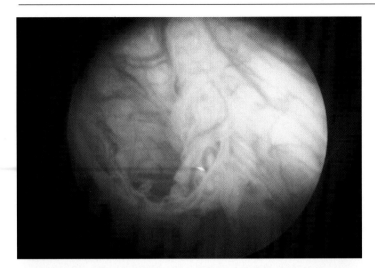

Figure 28.7 *Salpingoscopic grade IV: more extensive adhesions may be clearly seen (the normal fold pattern is totally disrupted).*

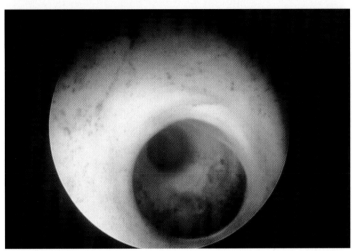

Figure 28.8 *Salpingoscopic grade V: complete loss of the mucosal fold pattern.*

Twenty-nine patients underwent salpingo-ovariolysis and 26 underwent salpingoneostomy. In all cases, tubal infertility was due to prior pelvic inflammatory disease. In the salpingo-ovariolysis group of patients, the term pregnancy rate was 66% (19/29), whereas for those patients with a normal ampullary mucosa (salpingoscopic grades I and II) this rate was 86% (19/22). In the salpingoneostomy group the term pregnancy rate was 31% (8/26) whereas for those patients with a normal ampullary mucosa it was 73% (8/11). At statistical analysis there was a significant correlation between salpingoscopic grade (grades I and II vs grades III to V) and the achievement of a term pregnancy for both the salpingo-ovariolysis and the salpingoneostomy groups of patients. There was no significant correlation between the AFS (American Fertility Society) score and the achievement of a term pregnancy for both groups of patients.

The use of salpingoscopy modifies the management of patients with tubal infertility, since accurate evaluation of the endosalpinx allows us to identify the patients with a normal tubal mucosa who may benefit the most from tubal reconstructive surgery (34–42% of cases of hydrosalpinx and 76–80% of cases of periadnexal adhesions). In these patients an intrauterine pregnancy rate ≥60% may be expected after salpingoneostomy and ≥70% after salpingo-ovariolysis. Hence, for such patients, reconstructive surgery should be the treatment of choice.

We also studied 18 patients in whom laparoscopy with tubal perfusion and salpingoscopy of the single remaining tube were performed for secondary infertility after contralateral salpingectomy for ectopic pregnancy. In all these patients, tubal perfusion revealed a patent tube. Salpingoscopy revealed a normal mucosal pattern in 13 of these patients. Eight of the 13 patients conceived an intrauterine pregnancy during the period of follow-up. In five patients, intra-ampullary adhesions were detected. In this latter group, three repeat ectopic pregnancies occurred during follow-up with one patient having first a term pregnancy and then a repeat ectopic. The proportion of patients who experienced a repeat ectopic was correlated with the presence of intra-ampullary adhesions at salpingoscopy but not with the presence of peritubal adhesions.

CONCLUSIONS

There is now growing evidence in the literature that the extent of intraluminal tubal damage does not necessarily correlate with the extent and nature of visible pelvic adhesions. In contrast there is a strong prognostic correlation between the status of the ampullary mucosa and the reproductive outcome of the patient.

SUGGESTED READING

Heylen SM, Brosens IA, Puttemans PJ: Clinical value and cumulative pregnancy rates following rigid salpingoscopy during laparoscopy for infertility. *Hum Reprod* 1995 **10**: 2913.

Marana R, Rizzi M, Muzii L, Catalano GF, Caruana P, Mancuso S: Correlation between the American Fertility Society classification of adnexal adhesions and distal tubal occlusion, salpingoscopy and reproductive outcome in tubal surgery. *Fertil Steril* 1995 **64**: 924.

Marana R, Muzii L, Rizzi M, Lucisano A, Dell'Acqua S, Mancuso S: Prognostic role of laparoscopic salpingoscopy of the only remaining tube after contralateral ectopic pregnancy. *Fertil Steril* 1995 **63**: 303.

Vasquez G, Boeckx W, Brosens I: No correlation between peritubal and mucosal adhesions in hydrosalpinges. *Fertil Steril* 1995 **64**: 1032.

29

FALLOPOSCOPY

Eric S. Surrey

Falloposcopy is an endoscopic approach for visualizing the lumen of the fallopian tube from the tubal ostium to the fimbria (Fig. 29.1). The procedure was first described by Kerin and colleagues. Candidates for this procedure include patients with suspected proximal or distal tubal occlusion by hysterosalpingo-graphy or by laparoscopic chromopertubation, those with unexplained infertility, and potentially those who are about to undergo tubal gamete or zygote transfer (GIFT or ZIFT). Falloposcopy should be performed after prophylactic antibiotic administration and during the mid-follicular phase of the menstrual cycle.

PROCEDURE

Two methods have been described: a coaxial and a linear everting catheter approach.

Coaxial approach

The coaxial method is derived from modification of well-established flow-directed cardiovascular access techniques. The patient is placed in low lithotomy position and a single toothed tenaculum is placed on the anterior lip of the cervix. The tubal ostium is initially visualized using a single operating channel flexible hysteroscope. A variety of instruments with a diameter (O.D.) ranging from 1.5–3.5 mm (Olympus Corp., Lake Success, NY; Mitsubishi Cable Industries,

Atamie, Japan; Intramed Laboratories, San Diego, CA) have been used. A camera attachment and a video monitor are used. A Tuohy-Borst Y connector (Cook Ob-Gyn, Spencer, IN) is attached to the operating channel. Ringer's lactate solution or embryo culture medium is used as distending medium. Culture medium is used if the procedure is being done prior to tubal gamete or zygote transfer. The hysteroscope is advanced to within 2 mm of the tubal ostium.

A floppy guidewire is then introduced through the second opening of the Y-connector (O.D. 0.3–0.8 mm; Conceptus Inc, San Carlos, CA; Guidewire Med-Tech, Watertown, NH; Cook Ob-Gyn). The material for the guidewire is Teflon or stainless-steel coated and platinum tipped. It is advanced into the tubal ostium under direct visualization using a gentle rotating motion. The guidewire should only be introduced when the ostium is clearly patent. Forced entry during an episode of spasm will induce bleeding. The wire is advanced to a distance of 12 cm or until resistance is met. In an effort to avoid perforation, further pressure should not be exerted at a point of resistance. Occasionally, it is necessary for an assistant to hold the tube with an atraumatic laparoscopic grasping forceps to facilitate the passage of the wire.

A flexible over-the-wire Teflon catheter (O.D. 1.2–1.3 mm; Conceptus Inc, Cook

Ob-Gyn; Target Therapeutics, San Jose, CA) with a second Tuohy-Borst Y connector attached to its proximal end is then introduced over the guidewire to a similar length (Fig. 29.2). The author has found that it is more convenient to introduce the guidewire and the catheter simultaneously with the guidewire extending 1 cm beyond the catheter tip. Once the guidewire has been properly positioned, the catheter is advanced further (Fig. 29.3).

The guidewire is then withdrawn and the falloposcope is introduced into the straight arm of the Y connector attached to the catheter (Fig. 29.4). Several flexible fallopo-

scopes with O.D. 0.35–0.5 mm and length 1.0–1.5 cm have been successfully used (Conceptus Inc, Olympus Corp.; Medical Dynamics, Englewood, CO; Intramed Laboratories). A second video monitor with a high resolution camera is used. Gentle gravity or pump infusion of Ringer's lactate solution or embryo culture medium through the second arm of the Y connector attached to the catheter is done to enhance visualization. Imaging is generally performed as the falloposcope and catheter are withdrawn to avoid a "white out" resulting from touching the walls of the fallopian tube. Recent investigation has centred

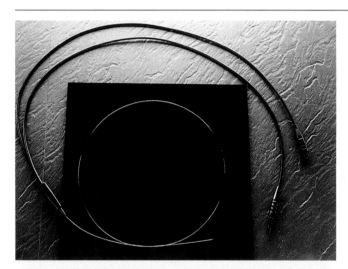

Figure 29.1 *Falloposcope (Conceptus, Inc., San Carlos, CA) with 0.4 mm O.D. and distal cameral attachment.*

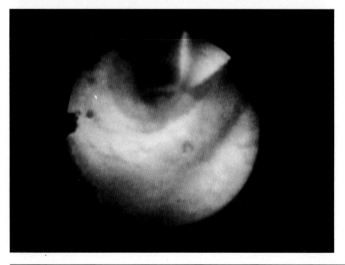

Figure 29.2 *Coaxial falloposcopy: falloposcope within outer catheter after successful tubal cannulation.*

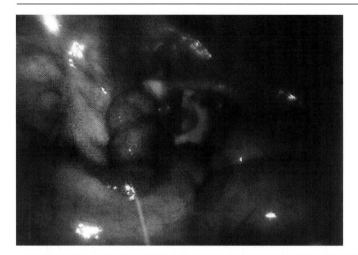

Figure 29.3 *Coaxial falloposcopy: laparoscopic view of guide wire extending through the fimbriated end of the fallopian tube and falloposcope at the ampullary-isthmic junction.*

around the development of an antegrade imaging system employing a protective wire shield around the catheter tip.

We found that placement of a moveable Mayo stand covered with sterile drapes between the patient's legs facilitates stabilization of the instruments and the elbows of the surgeon. Older devices require an assistant to stabilize the hysteroscope during the manipulation of the catheter, the guidewire and the falloposcope. A device attached to the operating table to hold the hysteroscope in place is currently under development. This will obviate the need for an assistant.

Linear eversion catheter method

An alternative means for performing falloposcopy is with the use of a linear everting catheter (LEC) (Imagyn, Laguna Niguel, CA) (Fig. 29.5). This unique system consists of inner and outer bodies joined by a distal balloon. As the balloon is inflated through an inflation port, the catheter tip everts. This allows the balloon to follow the course of the tubal lumen smoothly (Fig. 29.6). The falloposcope is introduced through the central lumen of the catheter. The tubal ostium is identified and after the catheter is fully everted, the tubal lumen is inspected. Ringer's lactate solution or embryo culture medium is gently infused through a third

port in the catheter (Fig. 29.5). Falloposcopy is performed in a retrograde fashion as the catheter is slowly withdrawn.

EQUIPMENT

For coaxial falloposcopy

1. Single tooth tenaculum, bivalved one-sided speculum
2. Flexible hysteroscope
3. Tuohy-Borst Y-connector (2)
4. Floppy platinum tipped guide wire
5. "Over-the-wire" Teflon-coated catheter
6. Falloposcope
7. Video monitor and camera attachments (2)
8. Extension tubing
9. Ringer's lactate solution or embryo culture medium infusion pump

For linear everting catheter falloposcopy

1. Single tooth tenaculum, bivalved one-sided speculum
2. Linear everting catheter
3. Falloposcope
4. Video monitor and camera attachments
5. Extension tubing
6. Ringer's lactate solution for embryo culture medium infusion pump

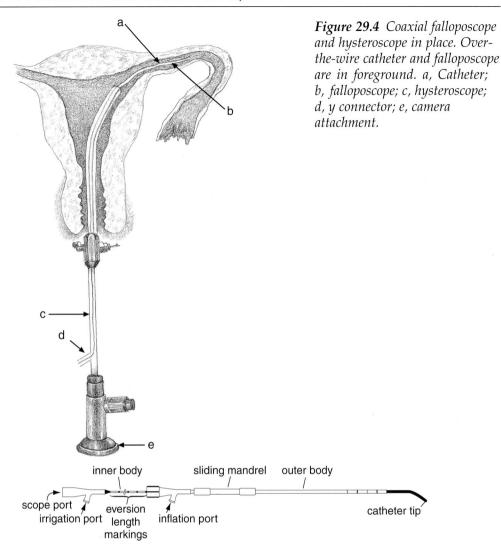

Figure 29.4 *Coaxial falloposcope and hysteroscope in place. Over-the-wire catheter and falloposcope are in foreground. a, Catheter; b, falloposcope; c, hysteroscope; d, y connector; e, camera attachment.*

inner body   sliding mandrel   outer body

scope port
irrigation port   eversion
length
markings   inflation port   catheter tip

Figure 29.5 *Linear everting catheter. Reprinted with permission from the American Society for Reproductive Medicine (Pearlstone A et al., Fertil Steril 1992 **58**: 854–857).*

ANAESTHESIA

When undertaken in conjunction with laparoscopy, falloposcopy is performed under general anaesthesia. However, several investigators have reported successful falloposcopy with a linear everting catheter employing local anaesthesia only. Coaxial falloposcopy may also be performed under conscious sedation particularly in conjunction with "micro-laparoscopy".

CLINICAL APPLICATIONS

The intramural portion of the fallopian tube is remarkable with the absence of mucosal folds (longitudinal rugae) whereas the isthmus tends to have four to six longitudinal folds (Fig. 29.7). The extent of primary and secondary folds increases towards the more distal aspects of the tube. A delicate vascular pattern can be identified (Figs 29.8 and 29.9). Various pathological findings have

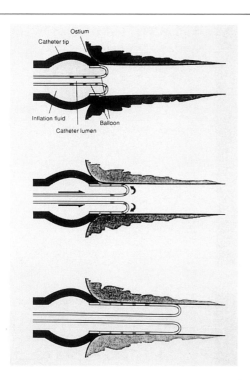

Figure 29.6 *Linear everting catheter: mechanism. Reprinted with permission from the American Society for Reproductive Medicine (Pearlstone A et al., Fertil Steril 1992 58: 854–857).*

been described including intraluminal mucus plugs, polyps, adhesions, varying degrees of stenosis, loss of vascular and architecture of the folds, and diverticuli compatible with salpingitis isthmica nodosa (Figs 29.10–29.13). A classification system attributing points for tubal patency, vascularity, epithelial pattern and extent of dilatation has been proposed by Kerin and coworkers. This system allows the surgeon to appropriately select patients for tubal reconstruction, intrauterine inseminations, gamete intrafallopian transfer, or tubal bypass with *in vitro* fertilization–embryo transfer.

Mucous plugs may be dispersed with gamete aqua-dissection. Stenosis and intraluminal adhesions may be approached with the passage of stiffer guidewires through the "over-the-wire" catheter or with introduction of a balloon catheter. Confirmation of tubal patency is obtained by performing follow-up falloposcopy. This approach allows the surgeon to diagnose the cause of tubal obstruction by direct visualization.

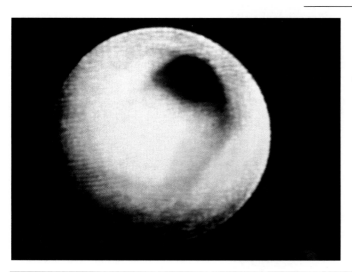

Figure 29.7 *Falloposcopic image of normal isthmus. Reprinted with permission from the American Society for Reproductive Medicine (Pearlstone A et al., Fertil Steril 1992 58: 854–857).*

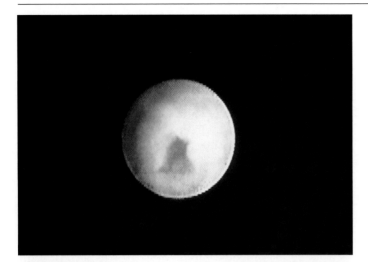

Figure 29.8 *Falloposcopic image of ampullary-isthmic junction.*

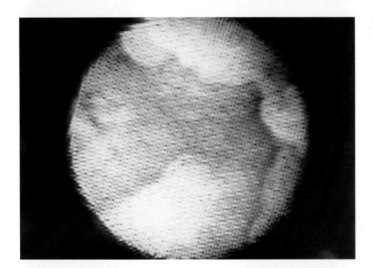

Figure 29.9 *Falloposcopic image of normal ampulla.*

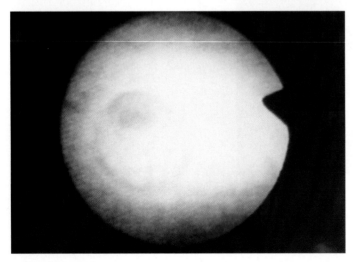

Figure 29.10 *Falloposcopic image of dense fibrotic obstruction at proximal isthmus.*

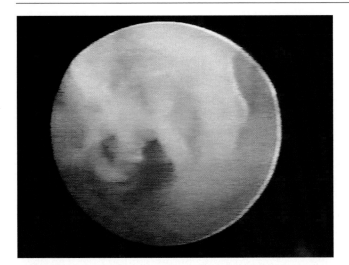

Figure 29.11 *Ampullary intraluminal adhesions.*

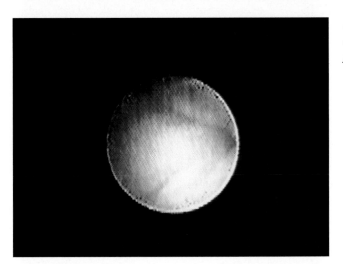

Figure 29.12 *Falloposcopic image of hydrosalpinx; note absence of mucosal folds or vascular patterns.*

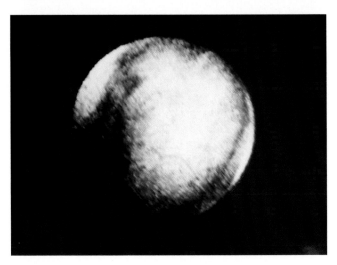

Figure 29.13 *Intraluminal polyp in mid isthmus. Reprinted with permission from the American Society for Reproductive Medicine (Kerin J et al.,* Fertil Steril 1992 **57**: 731).

POTENTIAL COMPLICATIONS AND THEIR PREVENTION

1. Inability to successfully advance the falloposcope or to visualize the tubal lumen adequately in the absence of any pathological findings has been reported in 8.5–13.4% of procedures. Clearly, the operator's experience plays a major role.
2. Tubal perforation without sequelae has been reported. The most common sites are at the uterotubal junction, the proximal isthmic region, the sites of tubal stenosis, and in the presence of peritubal or intraluminal adhesions. A low incidence of muscularis dissection by misplaced guidewires has been described. It appears that this is a minor complication not requiring any treatment.

CONTRAINDICATIONS

Falloposcopy is contraindicated in patients with acute or chronic genital tract infections. Patients with excessive or undiagnosed uterine bleeding are also poor candidates. Access to the tubal ostium may be difficult in patients with extensive submucosal or intramural leiomyoma in the cornual region.

SUGGESTED READING

Dunphy BL: Office falloposcopy assessment in proximal tubal disease. *Fertil Steril* 1994 **61**: 168–170.

Kerin J, Williams D, San Roman G, Pearlstone AC, Grundfest W, Surrey E: Falloposcopic classification and treatment of fallopian tube lumen disease. *Fertil Steril* 1992 **57**: 731–741.

Kerin J, Pearlstone A, Surrey E: Tubal microendoscopy: salpingoscopy and falloposcopy. In Keye WR Jr, Chang RJ, Rebar RW and Soules MD (eds) *Infertility: Evaluation and Treatment*. W.B. Saunders, Philadelphia, 1995, pp. 372–386.

Pearlstone AC, Surrey ES, Kerin JF: The linear everting catheter: a nonhysteroscopic, transvaginal technique for access and microendoscopy of the fallopian tube. *Fertil Steril* 1992 **58**: 854–857.

Scudamore IW, Dunphy BC, Cooke ID: Outpatient falloposcopy: intra-lumenal imaging of the fallopian tube by trans-uterine fiber-optic endoscopy as an outpatient procedure. *Br J Obstet Gynaecol* 1992 **99**: 829–835.

Surrey ES, Adamson G, Nagel T, Malo J, Surrey M, Jansen R, Molloy D: Introduction of a new coaxial falloposcopy system: a multicenter feasibility study. *J Am Assoc Gynecol Laparosc* 1997 **4**: 473–478.

30

ENDOSCOPIC FETOPLACENTAL SURGERY

Jan A. Deprest, Dominique Van Schoubroeck, Kamiel Vandenberghe and Yves Ville

Only a handful of life-threatening conditions for the fetus can be managed surgically during intrauterine life. Such procedures may either correct a congenital malformation, arrest the progression of a disease or temporarily alleviate a fetal condition until more definitive treatment after birth. Hysterotomy, irrespective of the procedure performed on the fetus, is a serious trigger for premature contractions and preterm delivery. It is hoped that an endoscopic approach may reduce postoperative uterine activity by minimal access and limit fetal morbidity by keeping the fetus within its natural environment. From a maternal viewpoint, this approach is also less invasive than laparotomy.

Fetoplacental endoscopic surgery is so far not a clinical achievement. Most if not all fetoscopic procedures are investigational, not validated and under debate. Patients should be counselled likewise, and follow-up must be very strict. Maternal safety must remain the primary concern. The procedures are delicate and should not be attempted without proper training. The endoscopic surgeon plays a temporary role in the ongoing care by the fetal medicine specialists. The ultimate patient is the fetus, surgically managed through the maternal abdominal wall. The invasiveness of the procedure is not measured by the number or diameter of the cannulas, but by the balance of an invasive procedure versus the improved fetal outcome.

EQUIPMENT FOR AND STAGES OF FETOSCOPIC PROCEDURES

Endoscopes, image display and distension medium

Key elements are the diameter, the length and the technology of the image transmission within the scope (fibreoptic versus rod lens). The smallest rod lens endoscope we used was a paediatric cystoscope with a diameter of 1.9 mm (Fig. 30.1). However, its length is not always sufficient to span the complete length of a polyhydramniotic cavity or to bridge maternal adiposity. We use fibre-endoscopes with diameters from 1.2 to 2.3 mm, and with the recent introduction of

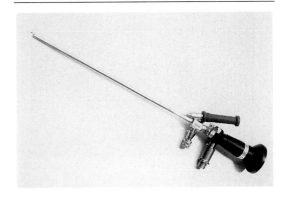

Figure 30.1 *0° rod lens fetoscope measuring 1.9 mm with sheath of 9.8 French.*

high resolution endoscopes (>30,000 pixels), image quality remains good even with endoscopes of 25–30 cm length (Fig. 30.2). Fibreoptics can be bent to a certain degree, which helps overcoming the absence of an angle of view.

The scopes are passed through operative sheaths; the diameter of which is usually expressed in French (3 French equals one millimeter). Instruments such as laser fibre, forceps or scissors can be inserted through the sheath. It can also be used for irrigation. During the procedure, ultrasound supplements the limited field of view of the fetoscope, and both endoscopic and sonographic images are simultaneously projected on the monitor (twin video system).

Contrary to laparoscopy, fetoscopy is performed in a liquid environment because of the concerns of adverse fetal metabolic side effects of CO_2. We use lactated Ringer's solution at 38.0 °C at minimal pressure. Amnion-irrigators are so far custom made. During the procedure the fluid balance has to be kept strictly, since intra-amniotic pressure directly affects fetal oxygenation.

Amniotic access and cannulas

The crucial point is to access the amniotic cavity safely and adequately, irrespective of how the maternal wall is penetrated. Depending on the surgeon, maternal incision can be merely a stab wound for a large needle or small cannula, or the uterus can be exposed partly through maternal laparotomy to insert trocars through the myometrium. The site of amniotic access is a compromise between the theoretical optimal cannula position and the limitations imposed by the actual fetoplacental position. For fetoscopic laser coagulation the scope can be inserted percutaneously and directed to the placenta (Fig. 30.3).

First the skin, abdominal wall muscles and the myometrium are infiltrated with local anaesthesia. The sheath loaded with a trocar is introduced under sonographic control. Low insertions are discouraged since they may increase the risk for amniotic leak or membrane rupture. In cases where the fetus, placenta or major uterine vessels hamper an anterior access, we suggest an "open" access, i.e. through a 2–3 cm mini-laparotomy and fundal, extraplacental cannulation (Figs 30.4 and 30.5). The myometrium is exposed and one can make a purse string to prevent amnion leak, or to arrest any haemorrhage after withdrawal of the cannula. However, it requires loco-regional or general anaesthesia, whereas the percutaneous technique is normally performed as a procedure under local anaesthesia.

When the sheath of the scope is not used as a cannula, other cannula types can be used. The diameter should be just large enough to accommodate the largest instrument. Cannulas should be relatively short to prevent overintroduction and soft tipped to

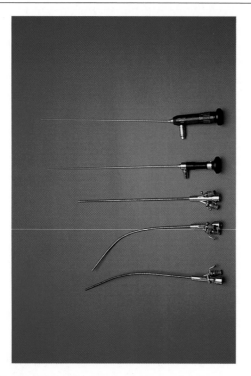

Figure 30.2 *(From top to bottom) 1.2 mm and 2.0 mm 0° fibrescope, with straight and bent sheaths, with a maximum outer diameter of 12 Fr.*

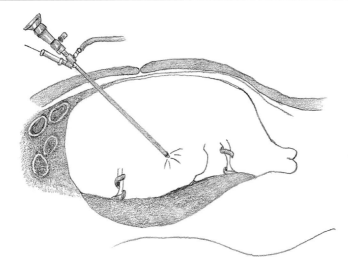

Figure 30.3 *Nd-YAG laser coagulation in case of a posterior placenta. The sheath of the scope has been used as a trocar, inserted percutaneously and directed at an optimal angle toward the intertwin membrane. Reprinted with permission of Parthenon Publishers from* Ultrasound in Obstetrics and Gynecology.

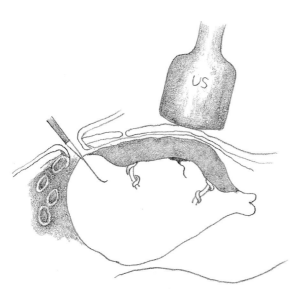

Figure 30.4 *Extraplacental approach through minilaparotomy, first step. Through a minilaparotomy bowels are retracted, and an amniocentesis needle is inserted. The needle is withdrawn, and a cannula and dilator are introduced over the guidewire. Reprinted with permission of Parthenon Publishers from* Ultrasound in Obstetrics and Gynecology.

prevent fetal trauma. To avoid unintentional withdrawal or membrane dislodgement they can be anchored to the abdominal wall. The ideal fetoscopic cannula is not yet marketed but we have used cannulas designed for vascular access, offering leakproof seal and a plastic side tubing for amnio-exchange. These come in any diameter, and are inserted by a Seldinger technique under ultrasound guidance. First an 18 G needle is inserted and a 0.085 inch (2.2 mm) soft J-tipped guidewire is introduced. The needle is removed and the cannula, loaded with a dilator, is advanced over the guide wire. The dilator gradually expands the myometrium to the diameter of the cannula, and thereafter the dilator and guide wire are withdrawn. At the end of the procedure a figure-of-eight suture of 2/0 polyglactin is placed through the myometrium. This stops bleeding from the uterine wall and leakage of amniotic fluid.

Special considerations

Patients receive prophylactic antibiotics, and tocolysis (we prefer indomethacin) for 48 hours. Some fetal conditions may

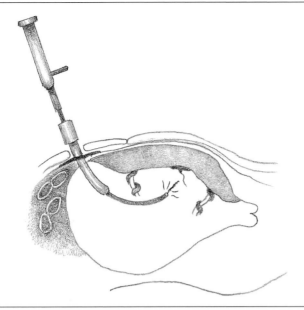

Figure 30.5 Trocar insertion technique, second step. The cannula has been fixed with a retention disc, and the bent fetoscope inserted, allowing full visualization of the intertwin membrane and the intertwin vessels. Reprinted with permission of Parthenon Publishers from Ultrasound in Obstetrics and Gynecology.

limit the prolonged use of indomethacin. Hospitalized patients are given low-molecular-weight heparin and carry varicose veins stockings. The fetus is monitored by ultrasound at 24 and 48 hours after the procedure. Further follow-up, medication or interventions, such as fetal transfusion, are decided according to the fetomaternal condition. Drinking, eating and ambulation are on patient demand.

POTENTIAL COMPLICATIONS AND THEIR PREVENTION

The exact nature and incidence of complications are not yet known.

1. Concerns about *in utero* exposure of the fetal retina to bright light. Animal data show that the fetal eyelids are protecting the fetal eyes. Before 26 weeks human fetal eyelids are closed.
2. The most common major complications are leakage of amniotic fluid and preterm premature rupture of the membranes (PPROM). Diagnostic fetoscopy is associated with a 3–5% PPROM-rate. A risk of 5–10% for PPROM is reported for fetoscopic laser coagulation, an operative procedure with only one cannula site. More complex procedures such as cord ligation have a 30% risk for PPROM prior to 32 weeks. Not only the number of cannula sites but also operation time or cannula diameter have been suggested as triggering factors.
3. Chorio-amnionitis and abruptio placentae.
4. Uterine wall haemorrhage at the cannula site may cause intra- or retroperitoneal and/or intra-amniotic bleeding. This impairs the fetoscopic visualization and may prevent continuation of the surgery. It may also prompt blood transfusion, which has more risks in pregnancy.
5. The haemodynamics of pregnant patients, particularly those under tocolytics and with fetoplacental hydrops predispose to pulmonary oedema. This is a theoretical consideration; no such case has yet been reported.
6. Fetal disease may also worsen the maternal status ("mirror" or maternal hydrops syndrome, where hydropic fetal symptoms are mimicked by the mother).
7. Direct fetal trauma by trocar insertion, instrumentation or the procedure are theoretical risks and should be avoidable by sono-endoscopic guidance of the procedure.

FETOSCOPIC Nd:YAG LASER TREATMENT FOR TWIN-TO-TWIN TRANSFUSION SYNDROME

Monochorionic twins have a three- to tenfold increased perinatal morbidity and mortality compared to dichorionic twins. This is due to the presence of functional placental vascular anastomoses between both fetal circulations (twin-to-twin transfusion syndrome, TTS). For years, active therapy has consisted in serial amniodrainages to reduce the polyhydramnios-related complications, such as preterm birth and maternal discomfort. Alternatively, fetoscopic Nd:YAG laser coagulation of anastomosing vessels can be done as a more "causal" therapy for severe TTS prior to 28 weeks gestation.

Diagnosis of monochorionic twins and its complications

The diagnosis of monochorionic twin gestation can be made with certainty by ultrasonography in the first trimester. A very thin midline septum between the two amniotic sacs can be seen, and a single extra-embryonic coelom with both yolk sacs. In the second trimester the diagnosis is based on the identification of fetal gender, the number of placental masses, and the intertwin membrane thickness. It is, however, less accurate. Sonographic evidence for TTS is the presence of a polyuric fetus surrounded by polyhydramnios (the recipient), and another (the donor) with no bladder filling and stuck to the placenta and uterine wall, tightly folded within its membranes (Fig. 30.6). The donor can be smaller.

Procedure

A 400–600-μm Nd:YAG laser fibre is passed through the operative channel of the fetoscope. Amnioinfusion may be needed to improve view or to clear the operative field from stained fluid, or abundant amniotic particles. The procedure can be done by minilaparotomy or percutaneously (Fig. 30.3). The polyhydramniotic sac is entered and the laser tip is inclinated as close as possible to a 90° angle towards the target vessels. Coagulation is done with power settings of 40–60 W at about 1 cm distance or less. Sections of approximately 1 cm are treated several times to ensure complete obliteration. The procedure is completed by amniodrainage until normal amniotic fluid levels.

Because of the difficulty in identifying arteriovenous anastomoses, Ville proposed coagulating all vessels crossing the intertwin membrane in order to separate the two

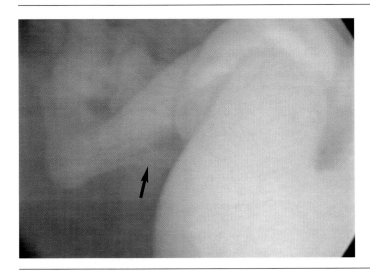

Figure 30.6 Fetoscopic image of a stuck twin. The membranes are draped around the legs and umbilical cord (arrow).

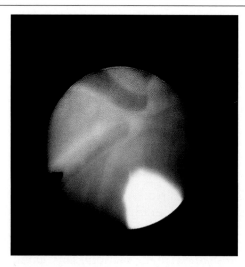

Figure 30.7 Superficial chorionic plate vessels cross the intertwin membrane. A 400-µm Nd:YAG laser fibre is used to coagulate vessels.

fetal circulations (Fig. 30.7). Although overtreating, the procedure is reproducible and fast because of its easy operative landmarks on the placenta.

Results and potential complications

After the procedure, about 75% of gestations end with the live birth of at least one twin. The overall fetal survival rate is about 55%. This matches the best results of serial amniodrainages. There is a much lower incidence of neurological handicap in the survivors (<5%) than reported for amniodrainage. This may be the most important incentive for the operation. A disadvantage of laser is the 25% fetal loss within a few days after surgery (usually of the donor). This is usually attributed to the non-selective coagulation of vessels not involved in the transfusion process. Other complications are those related to the amniotic access (PPROM), as well as incomplete lasering, persistence or reversal of fetofetal transfusion syndrome with fetal anaemia.

FETOSCOPIC CORD LIGATION

Acardiac twin pregnancy may be considered as the most extreme manifestation of TTS and complicates about 1% of monozygous twin pregnancies. In that situation a normal "pump" twin perfuses another abnormal fetus via reversed flow over an arterio-arterial anastomosis, connecting both umbilical cords ("Twin Reversed Arterial Perfusion"-sequence or TRAP-sequence). The umbilical vein of the parasitic fetus returns its deoxygenated blood directly into the placenta. The TRAP-sequence is associated with at least 50% mortality of the normal twin, mainly due to high-output cardiac failure or as a consequence of polyhydramnios and prematurity. The most logical treatment is to arrest the flow at the level of the umbilical cord of the abnormal twin. Cord obliteration can be achieved by ultrasound-guided cord embolization, fetoscopic cord coagulation or ligation. Fetoscopic cord coagulation with Nd:YAG laser is a procedure technically similar to chorionic vessel coagulation described above. It requires only one port. It fails however when the cord becomes too large and/or hydropic to allow effective coagulation, probably around 20–21 weeks. There is now some experience with bipolar coagulation of the umbilical cord, which has the advantage that it can be done through one port and completely under ultrasound guidance. It does not require sophisticated laser equipment and exceptional skills. Also, monopolar coagulation of major vessels in the fetus has occasionally been reported. Safety and performance of these techniques will have to be documented. Meanwhile, cord ligation is so far the most described technique.

Procedure

Fetoscopic cord ligation results in immediate, complete and permanent arterial and venous interruption of flow. The procedure is done with one or two ports (Figs 30.8, 30.9 and 30.10). In addition to the fetoscope,

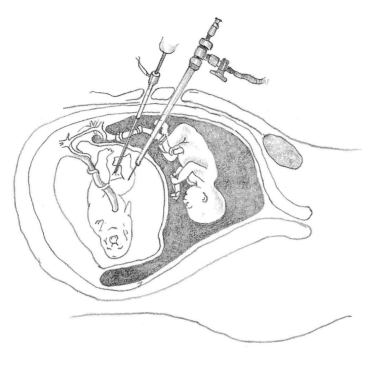

Figure 30.8 Technique of two-port fetoscopic cord ligation. The amniotic sac of the acardiac, laying under the placenta, has been opened. Instruments are inserted into that sac to do the actual procedure.
Amnioinfusion is by the scope, and drainage is done through the ports. Reprinted with permission from Deprest et al., (1997) Prenatal Diagnosis, Copyright John Wiley & Sons Ltd.

A   B   C

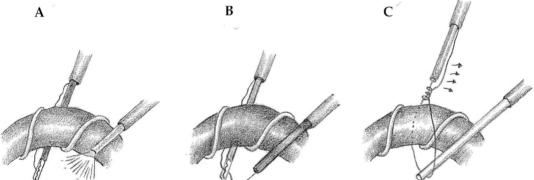

Figure 30.9 Steps in fetoscopic cord ligation. (A) Forceps brings suture behind the cord where (B) it is taken over by a second forceps inserted through the operative channel of the fetoscopic sheath. (C) When pulling out the suture end, or advancing the knot, tension on the cord by the suture material is avoided by supporting the material with the fetoscope or forceps. Reprinted with permission from Deprest et al., (1997) Prenatal Diagnosis, Copyright John Wiley & Sons Ltd.

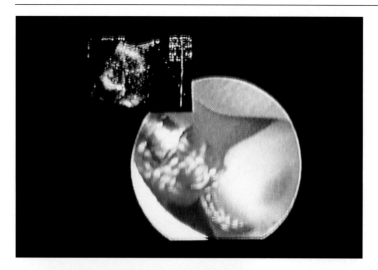

Figure 30.10 Fetoscopic cord ligation: fetoscopic view at the time of ligation. In the left upper corner, the projected ultrasonographic images are seen.

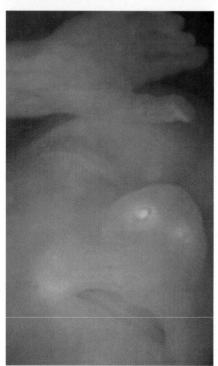

Figure 30.11 Fetoscopic image of a normal fetus.

one or two forceps and a knot pusher are used. One or two extracorporeal knots with a non-absorbable suture are made under combined ultrasound and fetoscopic guidance; the cord can be sectioned in between. The procedure is more complex than laser coagulation: of 23 attempted cases two failed because of haemorrhage or lack of workspace. Global fetal survival rate was 71% ($n = 15$). Striking is the occurrence of PPROM, about 30% before 32 weeks.

SUGGESTED READING

Adzick NS, Harrison MR: Fetal surgical therapy. *Lancet* 1994 **343**: 897–902.

Deprest J, Lerut T, Vandenberghe K: Endoscopic fetal surgery: a new perspective in fetal surgery? *Prenat Diagn* 1997 **17**: 1247–1260.

Deprest J, Van Ballaer PP, Evrard VA, Peers KHE, Spitz B, Steegers EA, Vandenberghe K: Fetoscopic cord ligation. *Eur J Obstet Gynecol Reprod Biol* 1998 (in press).

Luks FI, Deprest JA, Gillchrist BE, Peers KHE, van der Wildt B, Steegers EAP, Vandenberghe K: Access techniques in endoscopic fetal surgery. *Eur J Pediatr Surg* 1996 **6**: 1–4.

Ville Y, Hecher K, Gagnon A, Sebire N, Hyett J, Nicolaides K: Endoscopic laser coagulation in the management of severe twin-to-twin transfusion syndrome. *Br J Obstet Gynaecol* 1998 **105**: 446–453.

31

BASIC PRINCIPLES OF OPERATIVE HYSTEROSCOPY AND INSTRUMENTATION

Stephen L. Corson

The issues unique to operative hysteroscopy compared with diagnostic procedures basically resolve to two: the need for increased cervical dilatation to accommodate larger sheaths with operating instrument channels; and the problems created by violating the integrity of the endometrium, i.e. intravasation of medium and difficulties with visualization secondary to bleeding.

CERVICAL DILATATION

Cervical dilatation for diagnostic hysteroscopy is usually achieved by the telescope itself using carbon dioxide to distend the cervical canal and then the uterine body. When using a 3–5-mm instrument sheath, there usually is no need for prior passage of dilators. To the contrary, insertion of the telescope under direct vision is preferable to blind dilatation which may cause endocervical bleeding which will obscure visualization as the hysteroscopic lens passes these points. Operative hysteroscopy, on the other hand, may require dilatation to 11 mm in order to accommodate a resectoscopic sheath. Dilatation beyond 8 mm in a non-pregnant cervix frequently exceeds the elastic compliance of the tissue and actually tears the fibres. For that reason, we usually rely on a laminaria tent or an osmotic cervical dilator inserted into the cervical canal in the evening prior to morning surgery in order to achieve dilatation in an atraumatic and much easier fashion. Even if dilators must be used, the cervix has been partially dehydrated and yields more easily.

HYSTEROSCOPIC MEDIA

Although carbon dioxide is quite satisfactory to achieve uterine distension for diagnostic viewing and with minor operative procedures such as intrauterine device (IUD) removal and polypectomy, major procedures almost demand liquid media. Unlike laparoscopy, which is basically a closed system because absorption of gas from the peritoneal cavity is slow, the much smaller volume of the uterine cavity, especially when traumatized, can nevertheless absorb large quantities of gas and/or liquid rather quickly. In addition, the avenues of media egress through the fallopian tubes, outflow channel and cervix must be considered (Fig. 31.1). In order to achieve satisfactory uterine distension, a pressure within the cavity of the uterus of 45–80 mm of mmHg must be achieved. The flow rate necessary to reach this pressure is a function of the variables mentioned above. The pressure source with gas is usually an electronic hysteroscopic gas source (never laparoscopic) capable of delivering carbon dioxide

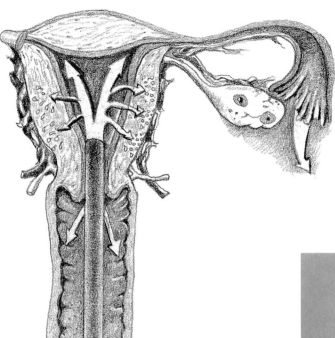

Figure 31.1 *Avenues of media egress from the uterus during hysteroscopy: fallopian tubes, outflow channel of the sheath, cervix, arterioles and venous systems.*

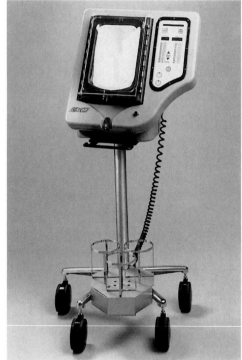

Figure 31.2 *A pump system to deliver liquid media during hysteroscopy at preselected pressures (the Dolphin™ CIRCON-ACMI).*

at higher pressure and less flow than for laparoscopy. Because of its solubility in blood, carbon dioxide is the only gas used for this purpose. Room air, even with inadvertent entry, can cause gas embolism. Liquid media are frequently delivered by gravity gradients, sometimes augmented with a pressure cuff, or by pumps which allow for preset and maintained pressures (Fig. 31.2). The single most important variable in pressure modulation is the outflow valve controlling the separate channel for return liquid. Although distension may be satisfactory, visualization may be compromised when the field is bloody. Therefore, the valve should be opened just enough to permit circulation of the medium sufficient for visualization. Even when intrauterine pressure is not excessive, high flow rates of electrolyte-free medium may cause hyponatraemia through the mechanism of membrane dialysis. An open vessel is a two-way street. Inadequate intrauterine pressure leads to a murky red field of view whereas excessive pressure causes intravasation leading to hypervolaemia (Fig. 31.3). Thus, when bleeding is encountered an intrauterine pressure equal to or just higher than mean arterial pressure is desirable.

The liquid medium of choice for operative

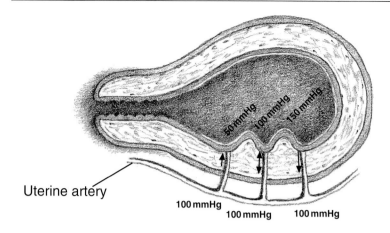

Figure 31.3 *Schematic diagram of uterine pressure versus mean arterial pressure (MAP) during hysteroscopy and intravasation.*

Uterine artery

hysteroscopy for many years was a solution of high molecular weight dextran. Its advantage is the feature of non-mixing with blood which greatly improves visualization. Although still used by a few surgeons, the disadvantages of cost, potential for allergic reactions, difficulty in delivery and increased instrument maintenance have dramatically lessened its use. Today the liquid media of choice for non-electrical procedures are physiological solutions such as saline or Ringer's lactate solution (never water, which will cause haemolysis) or dilute solutions of sorbitol or glycine when electrical current is employed. With use of electrodes capable of vaporization and high wattage settings, differences in electrosurgical generators have become more clinically important and attention to proper function of the dispersive electrode is mandatory.

LIGHT SOURCE

The light source must transmit through a properly maintained light cable sufficient light for both panoramic and close-up inspection. This usually translates to use of a xenon, halide or mercury vapour lamp rather than a simple halogen bulb. Although a 30° offset lens facilitates panoramic cavity inspection, most operative hysteroscopy

takes place in the centre of the area of view; consequently, operative telescopes are usually 12°–18° offset.

HYSTEROSCOPIC FORCEPS AND SCISSORS

Non-electrical procedures usually employ one of three types of forceps ranging from 7F to 9F diameter (Fig. 31.4). These are usually ridged graspers, biopsy forceps or scissors. In addition, an "optical scissors" (Fig. 31.5) fixed in place just ahead of the lens may be used to cut tough tissue such as fibrous adhesions or a uterine septum. Because these flexible or "semi rigid" instruments are long and narrow, mechanical advantage is limited, and even in gentle hands the cables and jaws break frequently. For that reason duplicates must be readily accessible. The hysteroscopic resectoscope differs little from the parent urological instrument (Fig. 31.6). Depending primarily on which electrode is inserted, coagulation, cutting or vaporization can be performed modulated by settings on the generator (Fig. 31.7). It is during these procedures of cutting as with myomectomy or entry into the myometrium during lysis of adhesions that significant intravasation of medium can occur, even at proper flow rate and pressure. As a consequence it is vital for the operator and nursing staff to have continuous, reliable data on the volume in and the volume recovered, since the difference – the deficit – represents the volume of fluid entering the patient, with a predominance of intravascular accumulation rather than intraperitoneal collection through the tubes.

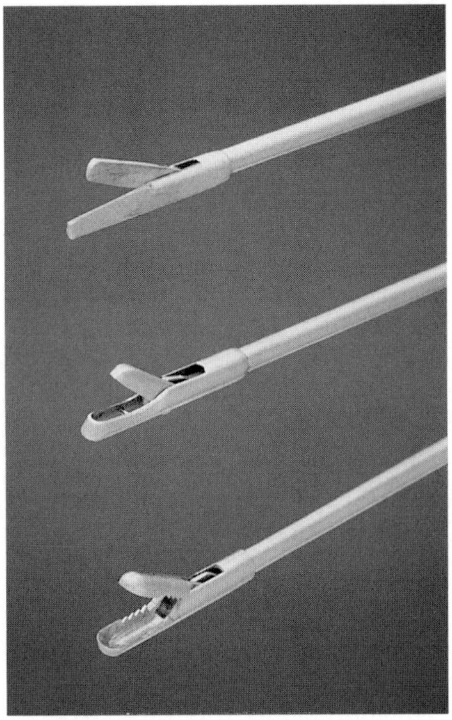

FLUID MEASUREMENT

Volumetric estimation of these fluids is inherently inaccurate. The 31 bags commonly employed have a ± 10% error factor as supplied by the manufacturer. Graduated fluid collection canisters are difficult to read accurately, especially in a darkened operating suite. To offset this, systems have been developed which measure by mass the inflow and outflow reservoir and which display the difference (Fig. 31.8). The proper placement of a fluid collection drape beneath the patient to collect outflow channel fluid and the liquid which has leaked out of the cervix is equally important. A helpful manoeuvre is to limit the amount of intravenous fluids given to the patient, especially if significant intravasation is a real risk. Depending on the size, age and cardiovascular status of the patient, intravasation of fluid up to 1000 ml can usually be safely tolerated. Beyond that, hyponatraemia and hypovolaemia may become a problem. The procedure should be quickly terminated at that point even if not completed and serum electrolytes measured. Therapy to correct imbalance includes use

Figure 31.4 Hysteroscopic ancillary operating forceps (from top): scissors; biopsy; graspers (CIRCON-ACMI).

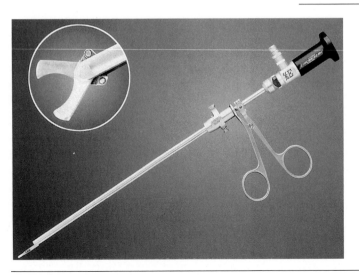

Figure 31.5 "Optical Scissors" for hysteroscopy (CIRCON-ACMI).

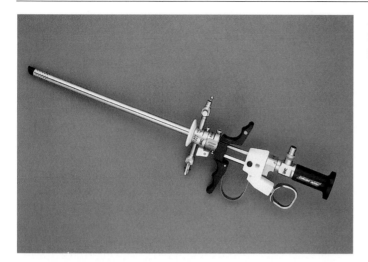

Figure 31.6 *Modern rotating inflow–outflow dual channel resectoscope (CIRCON-ACMI).*

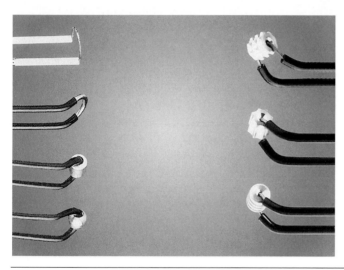

Figure 31.7 *Various electrosurgical elements used in hysteroscopy for cutting, coagulation and/or vaporization (CIRCON-ACMI).*

of intravenous furosemide and small amounts of hypertonic saline if serum sodium is dangerously low. Judicious use of dilute pitressin, 20 units/100 ml saline as a 2 or 3 ml injection into the cervical stroma (not submucosally) given at the commencement of the procedure reduces both operative bleeding and intravasation by the mechanisms of vessel spasm and myometrial contraction. This effect usually lasts for 15 or 20 minutes.

OFFICE HYSTEROSCOPY

As insurers and physicians have become more cost conscious, office systems have been designed to allow for basic operative procedures such as polypectomy, IUD removal, targeted biopsy and tubal cannulation, the latter frequently in conjunction with ultrasonic guidance. These systems function with both gas and liquid delivery systems (Fig. 31.9).

A surprising amount of surgery can be performed under paracervical block with or without supplemental intravenous sedation. Our protocol is as follows. First a wheal is made on the cervix with local anaesthesia at the point where the tenaculum is to be placed. Agents such as 1% mepivacaine or 0.25% bupivacaine without adrenaline are usually employed. Next,

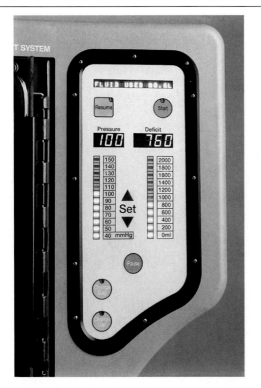

Figure 31.8 *Close-up of panel on Dolphin*^{TM} *System showing pressure and fluid deficit readings (CIRCON-ACMI).*

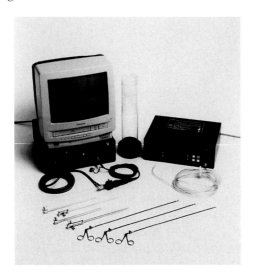

Figure 31.9 *Office hysteroscopy set – monitor-light source and gas source. Instrument soaker, wide-angle hysteroscope and camera with accessory sheaths for gas/liquid distension, and operating instruments (BEI).*

lateral traction is made with the tenaculum so that first one, and then the other, uterosacral ligament is put on stretch. The local agent is injected just beneath the cervical mucosa at the junction with the vaginal vault at the 5 and 7 o'clock positions. The volume is more important than the concentration of drug; 6–8 ml per side is used. A mild anaesthetic effect can be achieved with saline injection alone as a consequence of the pressure effect on the nerve endings. Bupivacaine gives a longer and deeper block but takes longer to achieve onset of action.

This anaesthetic protocol does not bring about any effect on the uterine fundus. Considerable surface anaesthetic effect can be obtained by infusing anaesthetic agent through the operating channel of the hysteroscope and keeping it in place for a few minutes (See Chapter 32). An intravenous cocktail of fentanyl and midazolam, approximately 75 mg and 2 mg, respectively, will give about 20 minutes of relaxation, pain relief, sedation and some amnesia. In the operating room propofol is frequently used instead.

CONCLUSIONS

Operative hysteroscopy has come of age. No longer must laparotomy and hysterotomy be performed for procedures within the uterine cavity. Endometrial ablation offers a viable alternative to hysterectomy for women suffering from menorrhagia. Although considered to be a "minor" outpatient procedure, complications of uterine perforation, excessive bleeding, fluid intravasation and room air embolism may cause considerable morbidity and even mortality. Safety starts with a well-educated operator using up-to-date equipment with proper technique.

SUGGESTED READING

Corson SL, Brooks PG: Resectoscopic myomectomy. *Fertil Steril* 1991 **55**: 1041.

Corson SL: Operative hysteroscopy for infertility. *Clin Obstet Gynecol* 1992 **35**: 229.

Corson SL, Brooks PG, Serden SP, Batzer FR, Gocial B: Effects of vasopressin administration during hysteroscopic surgery. *J Reprod Med* 1994 **39**: 419–423.

Corson SL, Brooks PG, Soderstrom R: Gynecologic endoscopic gas embolism. *Fertil Steril* 1996 **65**: 529–533.

32

OFFICE HYSTEROSCOPY

Carlo Romanini, Errico Zupi and Eugenio Solima

In the last few years there has been a growing interest in performing hysteroscopy as an office procedure. In order to be successful, it should be fast, easy to perform, with no excessive manipulation. With few exceptions, office hysteroscopy is mainly a diagnostic procedure. The advantages of office hysteroscopy include patient's preference, no special preoperative examinations needed and no requirement for general anaesthesia. The procedure takes several minutes with minimal amount of discomfort and the patient can observe the procedure by viewing the video-monitor. From the surgeon's point of view, this office procedure eliminates the nuisance of scheduling the patient in the operating room.

Diagnostic hysteroscopy has been historically compared to dilatation and curettage. Histological examination of hysterectomy specimens after curettage showed that in 60% of cases less than half the endometrium was removed with the curette and in 16% less than a quarter. The adequacy of curettage specimens collected for histological interpretation varies from 77% to 94%. The diagnostic value of hysteroscopy is attributed to its unique ability to investigate the entire uterine cavity enabling the observation of the shape, contour, relief, and colour of any pathology. Furthermore, a hysteroscopy-directed biopsy can be done if necessary.

INSTRUMENTATION

Hysteroscope

To carry out an adequate hysteroscopic examination and to perform office operative procedure a specific instrumentation is required. For diagnostic purposes, we prefer a rigid hysteroscope with a 30° lens allowing good visualization of the entire uterine cavity and the external sheath should be small enough to pass through the cervical canal easily (diameter 5 mm). Focusing ability allows the surgeon to come very close to the uterine wall for a "contact view".

Flexible scopes are also available. The flexibility enables easy access to the uterine horns and tubal ostia, but it gives less panoramic view than the rigid hysteroscopy.

Video camera, light source and hysteroflator

Cameras and light sources for laparoscopy can be used for hysteroscopic procedure. This has been discussed in Chapter 31. However, due to the risks of CO_2 embolism, the laparoscopic insufflator should never be used. Here, a hysteroflator is needed. This apparatus measures the flow rate and the intrauterine pressure. The flow rate can be preselected up to

100 ml/min. When it exceeds 200 mmHg the flow stops automatically.

DISTENDING MEDIA

Both CO_2 and saline solution have been described as safe distending media for office hysteroscopy. Carbon dioxide has the same refractive index as air and provides optimal clarity, but it needs a hysteroflator and it cannot be used in case of bleeding. CO_2 gas and blood produce bubbles which impair visualization. Here, low viscosity medium such as normal saline or solution of Ringer's lactate can be used. The advantages of such a solution are low cost, insufflation by a simple pressure bag, they are readily available and minimal risks of fluid overload. Also, blood clots and other debris are washed out with the liquid medium. A theoretical disadvantage is the need for a greater calibre of hysteroscopic sheath to allow fluid circulation in the uterine cavity and the inconvenience of fluid leakage. In our experience, hysteroscopy with CO_2 gas seems to be more painful than that with normal saline.

ANAESTHESIA FOR OFFICE HYSTEROSCOPY

It seems that paracervical block causes more pain than the hysteroscopy itself. We conducted a prospective randomized trial evaluating pain reduction during hysteroscopy and endometrial biopsy with local topical anaesthesia. In 45 patients, 5 ml of 2% mepivacaine or saline solution was injected transcervically into the uterine cavity before diagnostic hysteroscopy or a combined hysteroscopy and endometrial biopsy. Pain expectation and pain reported during and after the procedure were scored using a visual analogue scale. We found that instillation of anaesthetic agent into the uterine cavity reduces cervical pain and especially uterine pain during hysteroscopy and endometrial biopsy.

PROCEDURE

Minimal manipulation and swiftness of the examination are the key factors for a successful conduct of office hysteroscopy. Using these rules the surgeon can reduce the pain experienced by the patient, increase her compliance and allow better visualization of the uterine cavity. Pelvic examination and review of ultrasonography and/or hysterosalpingography results should be done before starting the procedure. In the presence of cervical stenosis or uterine prolapse, a tenaculum is placed on the anterior lip of the cervix to exert adequate counter-traction. Otherwise, we do not routinely use a tenaculum.

First, the hysteroscope and its sheath are gently inserted into the cervical canal under direct hysteroscopic control. In order to minimize cervical trauma, we recommend the following.

1. When using a 30° telescope, follow the canal by keeping "the dark area", represented by the cervical canal, at 6 o'clock on the screen.
2. When using CO_2 as distension medium follow the direction of air bubble or the flow of endocervical mucus.
3. Tubal ostia and lateral uterine wall can be evaluated just with slight rotation of the scope.

Usually, the hysteroscope can be inserted into the uterine cavity without any difficulty. In some cases of cervical stenosis (Fig. 32.1), transcervical injection of 2 mg mepivacaine into the uterine cavity will facilitate the procedure. Exploration begins with a panoramic view of the entire uterine cavity (Fig. 32.2) including its contour and the tubal ostia. The appearance of the endometrium depends on the time in the menstrual cycle (Figs 32.3–32.7). As the hysteroscope is withdrawn, the endocervical canal is reinspected. Most studies are completed in several minutes. If necessary a hysteroscopic directed biopsy is taken.

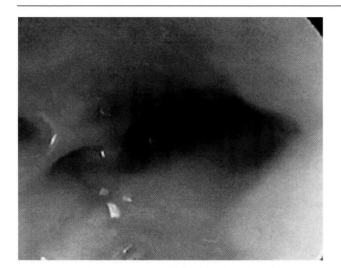

Figure 32.1 *A cervical stenosis is the most common cause of office-hysteroscopic failures.*

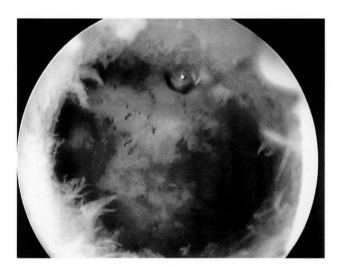

Figure 32.2 *A panoramic view of normal uterine cavity from the cervix. The circular wall of the cervical canal is white in appearance An air bubble is seen on the anterior wall. Courtesy of T. Tulandi M.D.*

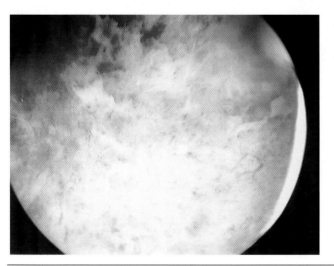

Figure 32.3 *Follicular phase endometrium. Courtesy of T. Tulandi M.D.*

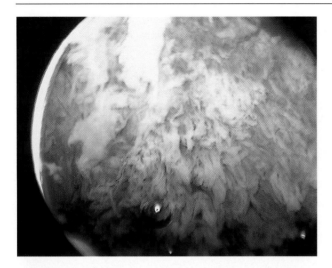

Figure 32.4. Secretory phase endometrium. Courtesy of T. Tulandi M.D.

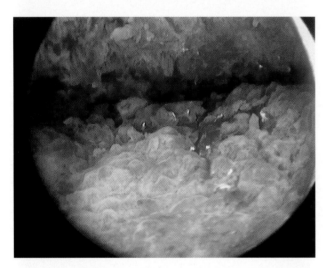

Figure 32.5 A thick secretory and polypoid endometrium. Courtesy of T. Tulandi M.D.

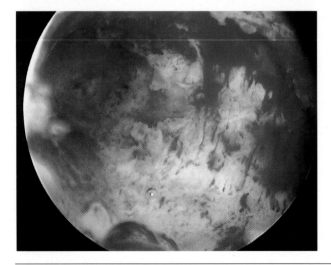

Figure 32.6 Endometrium on day 5 of menstrual cycle. Courtesy of T. Tulandi M.D.

INDICATIONS

The most common indications for office hysteroscopy are:

- Evaluation of an abnormal uterine bleeding (Fig. 32.8);
- To rule out an intrauterine cause of infertility;
- To locate and remove a lost intrauterine contraceptive device (Fig. 32.9);
- To evaluate the results of previous intrauterine therapeutic procedures;
- To verify endometrial sonographic irregularities and an abnormal hysterosalpingogram.

OFFICE OPERATIVE HYSTEROSCOPY

In addition to diagnostic purposes, diagnostic hysteroscopy can in some cases be extended to become a therapeutic hysteroscopy. This includes removal of an intrauterine foreign body, an endometrial polyp and a submucous myoma. Using a rigid hysteroscopic forceps inserted alongside the hysteroscope the foreign body is grasped and removed. A pedunculated myoma or polyp can be grasped and twisted, separating it from the uterine wall.

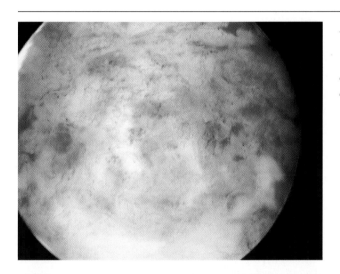

Figure 32.7 Atrophic endometrium 4 weeks after an administration of luteinizing hormone releasing hormone analogue (LHRHa), 3.75 mg of leuprolide acetate. Courtesy of T. Tulandi M.D.

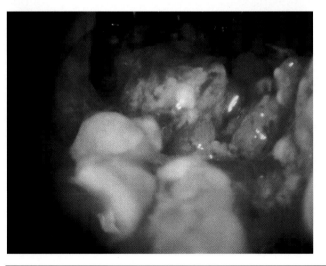

Figure 32.8 Endometrial cancer: a polymorphous thickened whitish endometrial surface is one of the most common hysteroscopic signs.

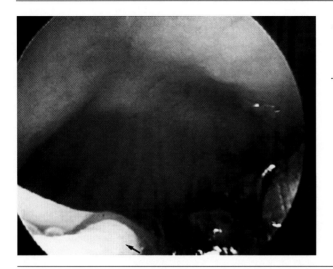

Figure 32.9 *A* lost *intrauterine contraceptive device* (arrow). *It can be removed easily using a hysteroscopic forceps.*

CONTRAINDICATIONS

No general consensus exists on contraindications to hysteroscopy. This is related to the rapid advances of hysteroscopic technology. Some of the contraindications discussed below may not be valid when smaller calibre scopes are used.

Pregnancy

Pregnancy should be ruled out before conducting hysteroscopy. In fact, in order to avoid poor visualization due to thick secretory endometrium, hysteroscopy is best done in early follicular phase of the menstrual cycle.

Endometrial cancer (Fig. 32.8)

Known uterine malignancy has been suggested as an absolute contraindication to hysteroscopy. It is believed that dissemination of endometrial cancer cells into the peritoneal cavity can occur during the hysteroscopy and prognosis can be impaired. However, Sugimoto performed hysteroscopy in 182 women with endometrial carcinoma with no apparent change in the prognosis. Tanizawa *et al.* showed that the number of endometrial cancer cells in the peritoneal cavity was not significantly dif-

ferent between women who underwent hysteroscopy and those who did not undergo hysteroscopy. Perhaps, this is due to the low intrauterine pressure employed in diagnostic hysteroscopy. Accordingly, the potential risk of peritoneal dissemination is minimized. Some authors consider hysteroscopic examination of the uterine cavity is an important step in the staging of endometrial cancer, defining the boundary between stages I and II.

Pelvic infections

Hysteroscopy should not be done in patients with salpingitis or possible salpingitis and in those with severe cervicovaginitis.

Cervical stenosis

This is a relative contraindication to office hysteroscopy. Cervical stenosis is found in less than 1% of cases. In most cases, cautious dilatation with curved and thin Kelly clamps resolves the problem. Also, insertion of a laminaria stent into the cervical canal a day before surgery will facilitate the procedure. However, it is often associated with overdilatation of the cervical canal causing gas or fluid leakage and subsequently insufficient uterine distension. We prefer to use transcervical injection of mepivacaine as described above. Alternatively, a half vaginal suppository of prostaglandin E2 can be inserted intracervically 30–45 min before the procedure. By using this technique, more than 80% of cervical stenosis can be resolved thus avoiding the need for general anaesthesia.

Cardiovascular disease

Cervical dilatation may cause a vasovagal reaction and bradycardia. Patients with cardiovascular disease, severe hypertension or asthma are best treated in the operating room where support personnel are available to handle these problems.

POSSIBLE COMPLICATIONS AND THEIR PREVENTION

The risks of office hysteroscopy are related to one of the aspects of the procedure: anaesthesia, uterine perforation and distension media. Accordingly, reducing anaesthesia may decrease complications. Another possible complication is vasovagal reaction. We found that in up to 4000 hysteroscopies less than 3% of cases experienced vasovagal reactions. They were mild and resolved in a few minutes. CO_2 gas has been associated with air embolism and occasionally death. These risks are eliminated by maintaining the insufflation pressure to below 100 mmHg. Although rare, uterine perforation and bleeding can also occur.

CONCLUSIONS

Hysteroscopy cannot measure angles and distances, so the surgeon's experience remains a very important factor in the interpretation of the hysteroscopic examination. The availability of a videotape recorder allows the operator to consult more experienced gynecologists after surgery. When in doubt, a hysteroscopy directed biopsy will establish the diagnosis.

SUGGESTED READING

Loffer FD: Hysteroscopy with selective endometrial sampling compared with D&C for abnormal uterine bleeding: the value of a negative hysteroscopic view. *Obstet Gynecol* 1989 **73**: 16–19.

Siegler AV: Hysteroscopy. *Obstet Gynecol Clin North Am* 1995 22(3).

Valli E, Zupi E, Montevecchi L, Solima E, Marconi D, Dini ML, Romanini C: A new hysteroscopic classification and nomenclature of endometrial lesions. *J Am Assoc Gynecol Laparosc* 1995 **2**: 279–283.

Zupi E, Luciano AA, Valli E, Marconi D, Maneschi F, Romanini C: The use of topical anesthesia in diagnostic hysteroscopy and endometrial biopsy. *Fertil Steril* 1995 **63**: 414–416.

33

HYSTEROSCOPIC LYSIS OF INTRAUTERINE ADHESION (ASHERMAN'S SYNDROME)

Robert S. Neuwirth

The term Asherman's syndrome is derived from the radiological description of filling defects in the uterus at the time of hysterography, in patients undergoing investigations for secondary amenorrhoea and/or infertility. Asherman first reported the relationship between endometrial trauma, curettage-associated with pregnancy loss or with postpartum haemorrhage, endometrial scar, and menstrual disorder and reproduction. The term Asherman's syndrome has become synonymous with intrauterine scar.

The diagnosis in the presence of amenorrhoea is established by ruling out a pregnancy if appropriate, administration of a progestin challenge, and finally an oestrogen challenge test with a high dose of oestrogen (5 mg Premarin daily for three weeks). Absence of menstrual flow following this treatment is diagnostic of absent or insensitive endometrium. Lower doses or shorter treatment is sometimes insufficient to elicit a response in a truly hypogonadotropic woman. Biphasic basal body temperature in the absence of menstruation is also usually diagnostic although I have seen rare instances of endometrial insensitivity as an exception to this rule. The diagnosis is definitively established by hysteroscopy. Hysterosalpingography is accurate if the uterine cavity is normal but only 85% accurate if filling defects are seen. Similarly, sonohysterography is a very accurate technique. In our institution, sonography in pregnancy has identified asymptomatic endometrial scars that subsequently were confirmed at Caesarean section or vaginal delivery. In order to enhance the accuracy of hysterographic or sonohysterographic techniques the fluid should be injected under videomonitor with controlled pressure of about 60 mmHg. This is to provide a gentle uniform distension of the endometrial cavity.

The treatment options vary from observation only to hysterotomy to break up the scar and reconstruct the endometrial cavity. Other options are blind scissors dissection and hysteroscopically controlled dissection. In younger patients with minimal disease the option of observation may be reasonable. In older patients or those with moderate or severe adhesions surgical repair is indicated if fertility is desired. Blind scissors dissection is unacceptable due to lack of precision and risk of injury. Open hysterotomy should be reserved for cases where the hysteroscopic approach is contraindicated or has failed and there is uncertainty if the plane of the endometrial cavity was ever identified. In such an instance a bivalve approach to the uterine fundus abdominally will establish the situation as well as give access to the residual endometrial cavity, if any. Sonographic and radiographic control of dissection may be complementary but not primary approaches.

The current technique of choice is the hysteroscopic approach. This should usually be done with a laparoscope in place unless the intrauterine adhesions are limited to distinct bands traversing the endometrial cavity. The adhesions can be simply divided and the bases will retract. As the endometrial cavity has only the tubal ostia and internal cervical os as landmarks the laparoscope adds to the safety of the operation. The pneumoperitoneum separates the uterus from the surrounding viscera in the event of perforation and the use of transillumination of the myometrium helps with safety and surgical orientation. Prophylactic antibiotics are routinely given just before surgery.

The method of dissection is preferentially with scissors (Fig. 33.1). The use of semirigid scissors may be preferable. Rigid scissors are fixed in front of the hysteroscope and may predispose to uterine perforation. Laser and electrosurgical methods can be used but depend on heat to accomplish the dissection and therefore produce some thermal damage adjacent to the line of dissection. Correlation with the hysterogram is extremely useful, especially in difficult cases, to determine the anatomy (Figs 33.2–33.6). At times after dissection is started and the adhesions are not dense the use of a blunt curette and ovum forceps,

opening them gently in the endometrial cavity, will expedite the dissection. Sometimes, filmy and thin adhesions can be disrupted simply by inserting the hysteroscopic sheath.

After dissection the cavity should be measured longitudinally and transversely and recorded. In infertile patients, the fallopian tubes should be inspected and chromopertubation using indigo carmine performed. Failure to demonstrate patency is not necessarily a diagnosis of tubal obstruction as debris and clot may block dye passage at this time. The dye may infiltrate the myometrium and give evidence of the extent and depth of the dissection within the uterine body and help determine the adequacy of the surgery. Transillumination with the laparoscope light extinguished will also help to determine the adequacy of the dissection. An unusually bright light inside the uterine cavity indicates thin uterine wall and dissection on that particular area should be discontinued.

At the end of the procedure a splint is used. A non-medicated plastic IUD can be inserted, or a Foley catheter, or custom made silastic rubber balloon stent. The splint is left in place for one week and oestrogen (Premarin 1.25 mg q.i.d.) is given for two 21-day courses. It is our practice not to add a progestin at the end of the courses

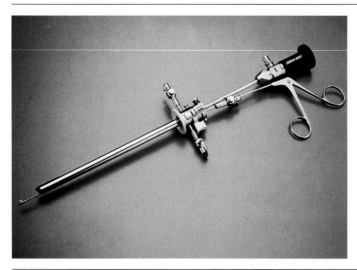

Figure 33.1 An operative laparoscope with scissors in place. Note the short working distance between the objective of the lens and the tip of the scissors that can distort the image during surgery.

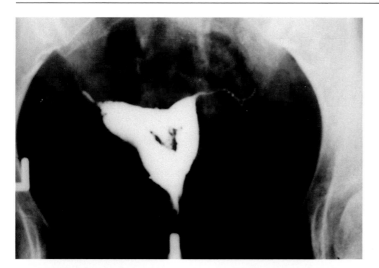

Figure 33.2 Preoperative hysterogram in a patient with secondary amenorrhoea revealing a central scar.

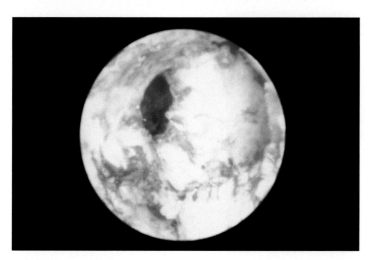

Figure 33.3 Inferior aspect of the scar from a patient described in Figure 33.2. Note channels on either side of the scar confirming the hysterographic findings.

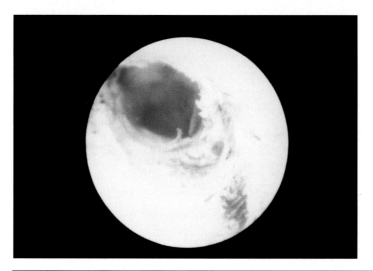

Figure 33.4 Lower margin of the scar from the same patient. The small entry into the channel on the left side of the scar indicates the location to start the dissection.

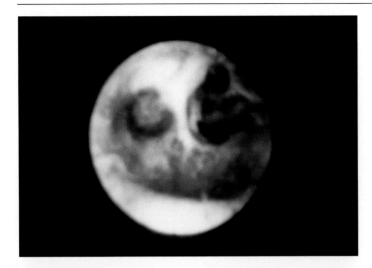

Figure 33.5 Badly scarred uterine cavity with thick bands and scattered foci of endometrium. Tubal ostia are not seen.

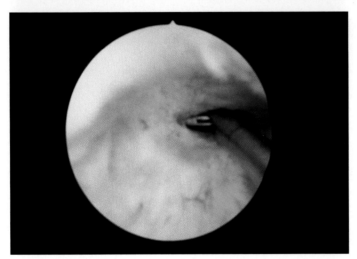

Figure 33.6 Scissor dissection is started.

as the purpose of oestrogen is to hyperstimulate endometrial proliferation only.

In our experience with 195 cases, restoration or improvement of menstrual function is approximately 90%. Persistent amenorrhoea is generally found in those patients who had total obliteration of the endometrial cavity at the time of the hysteroscopic exploration. There are several notable exceptions where a normal cavity, menstrual function and successful reproduction resulted following repair in the severe group. In patients with areas of normal endometrium seen at preoperative hysteroscopy or hysterography, all of them resumed some menstrual function or returned to normal menses. In addition, the endometrial cavity was restored to normal at the postoperative hysterogram. Successful pregnancies are reported in about 80% of cases. In our series, conception occurred in 55 of 103 cases followed-up for a year.

COMPLICATIONS AND THEIR PREVENTION

1. Uterine perforation. The complications in our series have been limited to uterine perforation which occured in 11 cases. No bowel injury occurred and the consequence has been to terminate the proce-

dure when the perforation prevented uterine distension. The operation was completed two months later. Concomitant laparoscopy has been used in all cases where the scar bands blended into the wall of the endometrial cavity. Uterine perforation was detected early and there was no injury to adjacent viscera.

2. Bleeding and infection. There has been no haemorrhage requiring transfusion and no infection has been seen. Because the normal anatomy is usually distorted, dissection must be kept in the endometrial cavity. Deviation can lead to perforation, or vascular injury if lateral and below the broad ligament. It can also damage large arteries and veins near the serosa predisposing to serious haemorrhage. If large venous channels are cut, the risk of fluid overload is higher.

3. Fluid overload. Fluid overload has not been seen and is avoided by careful attention to fluid balances. The vast majority of patients have been treated with Hyskon as the distending medium. Hyskon is usually chosen for these cases because the cavity is frequently small. Also, the operative field is not perturbed by the flow which is seen with low viscosity, continuous flow hysteroscopy. However, in order to avoid sticking of scissors and valves due to Hyskon, the instruments must be washed carefully and promptly after their use.

4. Placenta accreta. This complication has been seen after treatment of moderate and severe intrauterine adhesions.

CONTRAINDICATIONS

Patients with severe liver, cardiac or renal disease are not candidates for a long hysteroscopic procedure. They are at risk for fluid overload and electrolytes imbalance. The complications of hysteroscopic lysis of adhesions are rare when the surgery is performed skillfully and prudently. The outcome is good for menstrual function and fair for reproductive outcome.

SUGGESTED READING

Asherman JG: Amenorrhea traumautica (atretica). *J Obstet Gynaecol Br Emp* 1948 **55**: 23–27.

Ferenczy A: Studies on the cytodynamics of human endometrial regeneration. II Transmission electron microscopy and histochemistry. *Am J Obstet Gynecol* 1976 **28**: 582–595.

March CM, Israel R, March, AD: Hysteroscopic management of intrauterine adhesions. *Am J Obstet Gynecol* 1978 **130**: 653–657.

Polishuck WZ, Adoni A, Aviad I: Intrauterine device in the treatment of traumatic intrauterine adhesions. *Fertil Steril* 1969 **20**: 241–249.

34

HYSTEROSCOPIC POLYPECTOMY AND MYOMECTOMY

Togas Tulandi

HYSTEROSCOPIC POLYPECTOMY

During the investigations of abnormal uterine bleeding, a dilatation and curettage (D&C) is often done. However, D&C is a blind procedure and up to 25% of the endometrium is missed by this procedure. An endometrial polyp is also often missed. Hysteroscopy is invaluable in the management of abnormal uterine bleeding. Preoperative investigations include transvaginal ultrasonography or preferably a hysterosonogram to detect an intrauterine lesion. The patient can then undergo an operative hysteroscopy. Hysteroscopy is performed to establish the diagnosis and also for treatment.

Hysteroscopy is best done a few days after menstruation or after preoperative treatment with a single dose of long-acting depot LHRHa (luteinizing hormone releasing hormone analogue). We use leuprolide acetate 3.75 mg intramuscularly in the mid-luteal phase and hysteroscopy is done 4 weeks after the injection. The thin endometrium allows visualization of the uterine cavity without interference from thick secretory endometrium.

PROCEDURE

Under general or spinal anaesthesia, the cervix is first dilated up to 9 mm. The resectoscope is inserted into the uterine cavity and using glycine 1.5% as a distending medium, the uterine cavity is evaluated systematically (Fig. 34.1). An endometrial polyp is easily diagnosed by its reddish appearance similar to the surrounding endometrium (Fig. 34.2). Usually, it has a broad base and is soft. Contrary to a myoma, it moves with the movement of the distending solution. The base of the polyp can be cut with a 90° loop electrode. The loop is placed behind the polyp and it is retracted from the direction of the uterine fundus towards the cervix. This is to avoid uterine perforation. It is crucial that the electrode is seen all the time. A larger polyp can be shaved to its base (Fig. 34.3). A cutting current with a unipolar mode at 80–100 W is used. Bleeding points are coagulated with light application of the loop electrode using coagulating current at 40 W. A polyp attached at the end of the loop can be extracted by removing the instrument. Otherwise, it is removed with a blunt curette or a forceps.

Another technique is to encircle the polyp with a retractable unipolar snare loop. The snare is inserted through a 3-mm operating channel of a multichannel operating hysteroscope. The loop is tightened around the base of the polyp and the polyp is cut with 40 W cutting current. A solitary polyp or myoma of less than 1 cm can be removed under local or paracervical block anaesthesia.

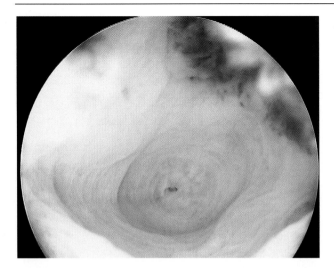

Figure 34.1 A close-up view of right tubal ostium.

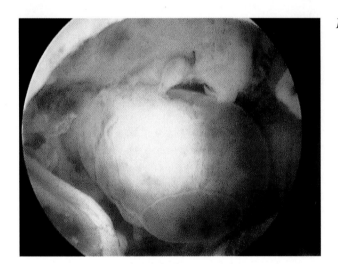

Figure 34.2 An endometrial polyp.

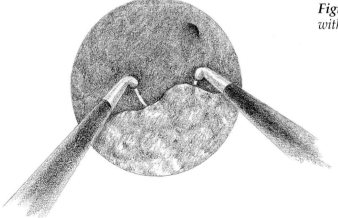

Figure 34.3 Excising a broad-based polyp with a 90° loop electrode.

HYSTEROSCOPIC MYOMECTOMY

A submucous myoma is excised in a similar manner to hysteroscopic polypectomy. Hysteroscopic myomectomy is facilitated by thinning the endometrium with at least one dose of long-acting LHRHa. Longer duration of LHRHa treatment (3 months) is indicated if the submucous myoma is > 5 cm. LHRHa decreases the size of the myoma and its vascularity. Maximal shrinkage is obtained after 3 months of treatment. Another advantage of preoperative treatment with LHRHa is the improvement of the patient's haematological status.

PROCEDURE

In the presence of multiple submucous myomas, it is advisable to start with the smaller one that is located closest to the cervical os. This is to avoid fragments of resected myoma obscuring visibility. Also, anterior myoma should be excised first as air bubbles tend to accumulate anteriorly. The myoma fragments are pushed into the uterine fundus instead of removing each fragment. Excision is done repeatedly until the myoma is completely removed, usually until the level of myometrium. This is indicated by the changing appearance of pale fibrous tissue to striated myometrium. The

surface defect tends to heal without scar formation. Cutting is done by moving the loop in and out by a hand mechanism of the resectoscope. It can also be done by moving the whole resectoscope outward with the loop extended. Myomas can be excised with the use of a 90° loop electrode (Fig. 34.4). However, this may be difficult for a fundally located myoma. Here, the angle of the loop can be increased to 135°. The position and the angle of the instrument against the uterus play an important role in the conduct of operative hysteroscopy. At the completion of the cutting phase, the myoma fragments are removed using a blunt curette or forceps. The remaining fragments will be expelled spontaneously in a few days.

A large myoma can be separated from the uterine wall by cutting its base until the myoma is floating free in the uterine cavity. The size is reduced by incising it with the loop electrode or it can be left in the uterine cavity for spontaneous expulsion in a few days. Usually, a jelly like structure is passed without any discomfort. A newly developed vaportrode is another alternative. At 200°, it can "melt" the myoma. Cutting the cervix to facilitate removal of a large specimen is unnecessary.

A prolapsed pedunculated submucous myoma can be twisted off. However, a

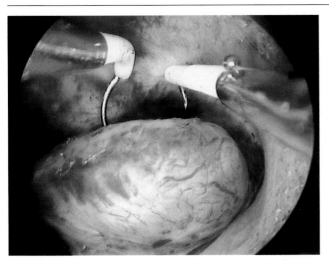

Figure 34.4 Hysteroscopic myomectomy. A loop electrode is placed behind the myoma and retracted outward from the direction of the uterine fundus toward the cervix.

broad pedicle is better sutured or tied first with absorbable suture material. The myoma distal to the pedicle is then cut. The pedicle itself will retract and does not need further removal.

COMPLICATIONS AND THEIR PREVENTION

1. Cervical tear can occur during difficult cervical dilatation and during hysteroscopic procedure. If the cervix is stenotic, a laminaria stent can be inserted several hours before surgery. This is rarely needed.
2. Uterine perforation and injury to intra-abdominal organs with an electrode is avoided by cutting from the direction of uterine fundus toward the cervix. The greatest risk of perforation tends to occur during excision of a central fundal myoma. When there is concern about perforation, a concomitant laparoscopy should be done. Trauma to iliac vessels can occur as a result of uterine perforation.
3. Infection and bleeding after hysteroscopic procedures can occur, but they are rarely encountered. Hysteroscopy should not be done in the presence of pelvic inflammatory disease or when it is suspected.
4. Bleeding can be encountered during removal of a broad-base myoma. Bleeding points should be coagulated with coagulating current. Persistent bleeding from the base of the myoma may need tamponade. This is done by inserting a Foley catheter into the uterine cavity and the balloon is inflated to 30 ml. The catheter is removed after 24 hours.
5. One of the most important complications of operative hysteroscopy using low viscosity solution is fluid overload or severe electrolyte imbalance. This can lead to brain oedema and death. Close attention to fluid intake and output is mandatory. If the deficit is ≥ 1000 ml, intravenous injection of 10 mg of frusemide is recommended. Fluid deficit of >1500 ml during the procedure should be followed by termination of the procedure. This may be the case during resection of a large myoma. A repeat myomectomy can be arranged at a future date.

CONTRAINDICATIONS

Several criteria have to be met before performing hysteroscopic myomectomy. A large uterine cavity cannot be distended adequately with the distending medium, accordingly the uterine depth should be less than 10 cm. The myoma should be <5 cm and more than half of the myoma should be located in the uterine cavity. Patients with severe liver, cardiac or renal disease are not candidates for a long hysteroscopic procedure. They are at risk for fluid overload and electrolyte imbalance. Hysteroscopy should not be done in the presence of pelvic inflammatory disease or when it is suspected.

SUGGESTED READING

Valle RF: Hysteroscopic evaluation of patients with abnormal uterine bleeding. *Surg Obstet Gynecol* 1981 **153**: 521.

Neuwirth RS: Hysteroscopic submucous myomectomy. In *Infertil Reprod Med Clin North Am* 1996 **7**: 91–108.

35

ENDOMETRIAL ABLATION

Roger Hart and Adam Magos

Endometrial ablation encompasses several techniques designed to reduce menstrual blood loss as an alternative to hysterectomy for the management of abnormal bleeding of benign origin. Loop electrosurgical resection, electrosurgical rollerball and laser ablation are the commonest techniques employed. Recently some even less invasive techniques have been developed but these are still in the evaluation phase.

TRANSCERVICAL ENDOMETRIAL RESECTION (TCRE)

The development of the intrauterine resection of submucous fibroids by Neuwirth in 1978 was the first use of the urological resectoscope in the uterine cavity leading to its adaptation to treat the whole endometrial cavity with TCRE.

Instrumentation and preoperative preparation

The equipment commonly used are a 26 French gauge continuous flow passive handle resectoscope with a 4-mm forward oblique endoscope and a 24 French gauge cutting loop. The use of a passive handle mechanism ensures that the cutting loop is inside the sheath at rest and consequently accidental trauma is unlikely. Distension of the uterine cavity for adequate visualization

of the fundus is achieved by using an irrigation pump to maintain an intrauterine pressure of 80–120 mmHg. Insufficient intrauterine pressure provides inadequate uterine distension and overdistension can lead to problems of excessive fluid absorption. To maintain a continuous flow of uterine irrigant, a suction device is attached to the outflow of the resectoscope to generate a negative pressure of around 50 mmHg. The suction pressure may be increased if the view is too cloudy, or decreased if uterine distension is inadequate prior to increasing the distension pressure. The distension media commonly used is 1.5% glycine although other non-conductive media can be used.

Prior counselling ensures that the patient has completed her family, has menorrhagia sufficient to warrant surgery and understands the remote possibility of the procedure converting to a hysterectomy. The best results from TCRE are obtained where uterine size is less than the equivalent of a 12 weeks gestation, where there are not too many submucous fibroids and where the woman has received endometrial preparation. The use of gonadotrophin releasing hormone analogues (GnRH) or danazol for six weeks prior to the surgery ensures that the endometrial thickness is no greater than 3 mm, which facilitates resection of the endometrium and superficial myometrium.

Procedure

The procedure may be performed under general or local anaesthesia. If local anaesthesia is used premedication of a benzodiazepine is given combined with peroperative sedation with intravenous midazolam. Local anaesthetic block is provided by intracervical, paracervical and intrauterine lignocaine with adrenaline, and additional analgesia is obtained by small intravenous doses of an opioid such as fentanyl.

The cervix is first dilated incrementally to a size 10 Hegar dilator. A blended cutting and coagulation current is used to produce cutting with haemostasis (e.g. 100–120 W). Any submucous fibroids are usually resected first particularly if they obscure parts of the uterine cavity. Next, the uterine fundus is treated using either a forward-angled loop to resect the endometrium or a rollerball to ablate it (Figs 35.1–35.4). The rest of the uterus is resected with the conventional loop in a systematic manner down to the internal os (Figs 35.5–35.8). The depth of resection is judged by the appearance of the circular myometrial fibres (Fig. 35. 9), and it is important not to cut too deep as this could lead to haemorrhage and ultimately uterine perforation. The resected tissue chips can be pushed towards the fundus to enable visualization of the unresected part of the endometrial cavity (Fig. 35.10), and only removed at the end the procedure, using a flushing curette. This is our preferred technique, but when the endometrium is thick it is sometimes easier to cut full length chips which are removed from the uterine cavity with each pass of the resectoscope. At the end of the procedure, the uterus is reinspected to ensure the resection is complete (Figs 35.11 and 35.12) and that there are no bleeding vessels. Any obvious bleeding points can be cauterized using 60 W of coagulation current. Generalized bleeding can be controlled by inflating the 30 ml balloon of a urinary catheter inside the uterine cavity to cause tamponade.

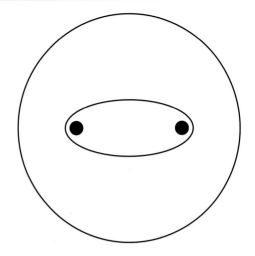

Figure 35.1 *The normal endometrial cavity with the ostia visualized prior to endometrial resection.*

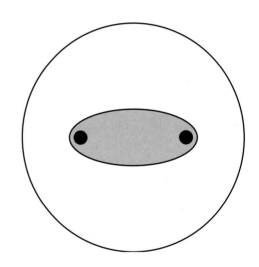

Figure 35.2 *The fundus is treated first with either the forward angle loop or the rollerball.*

Results

O'Connor and Magos in 1996 reported on the follow-up of patients undergoing endometrial resection for up to 5 years using life-table analysis. It was found that 26–40% of women reported amenorrhoea, 71–80% noted an absence or amelioration of their dysmenorrhoea, and 79–87% were

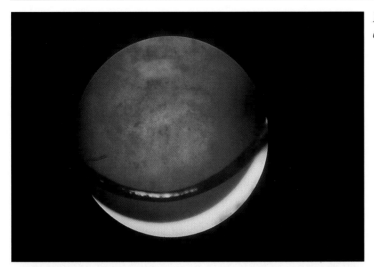

Figure 35.3 *The forward pointing electrosurgical loop.*

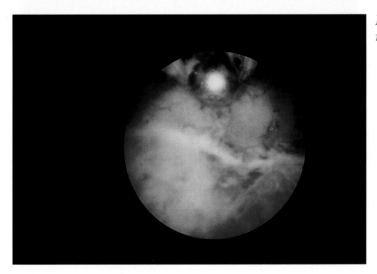

Figure 35.4 *Applying the rollerball to the endometrium.*

satisfied with their treatment. About 3% of women were given medical therapy for recurrent symptoms and 16% required further surgery. Ultimately, 9% of women underwent hysterectomy for heavy, painful periods or pelvic pain. Life-table analysis showed that 80% of women avoided further surgery and 91% avoided hysterectomy during the 5 years after their surgery.

Complications and their prevention

1. Fluid overload. It is very important that fluid balance is strictly monitored preop-eratively to avoid the complications of fluid overload which is associated with hyponatraemia and encephalopathy if a low viscosity solution is used as the distension medium. Surgery should be stopped and intravenous diuretics administered if the fluid absorbed is greater than 1500 ml.

2. Uterine perforation. Common problems during endometrial resection or ablation are those related to uterine distension. The inflow pressure largely controls uterine distension, but if distension is suddenly lost the surgeon must exclude uterine perforation. Similarly, the pressure

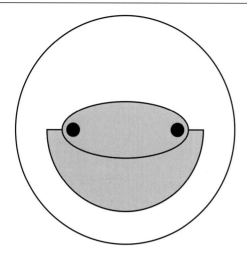

Figure 35.5 *The upper posterior part of the endometrial cavity is treated first.*

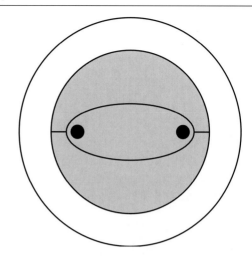

Figure 35.6 *Now treating the anterior wall.*

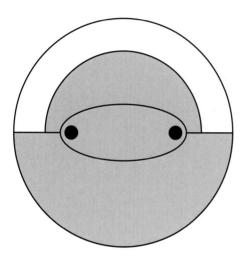

Figure 35.7 *Then the posterior wall of the uterine cavity is completed.*

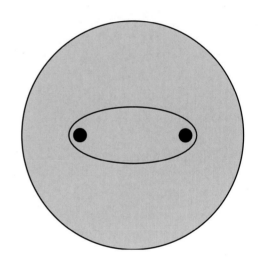

Figure 35.8 *The anterior wall is completed.*

in the uterus should not exceed 120–150 mmHg as the patient will run the risk of rapid fluid absorption. If the field of view becomes cloudy, the negative pressure generated by the suction equipment can be increased to remove debris from the field of view. Uterine perforation occurs in up to 4% of cases overall, but can be as high as 8% with repeat pro-

cedures. If the perforation occurs with an activated resectoscope, a laparoscopy or laparotomy is mandatory to ensure no adjacent viscus has been lacerated.
3. Haematometra. The development of haematometra due to unresected fundal islands of endometrial tissue is not an infrequent complication and can be treated by performing a repeat resection.

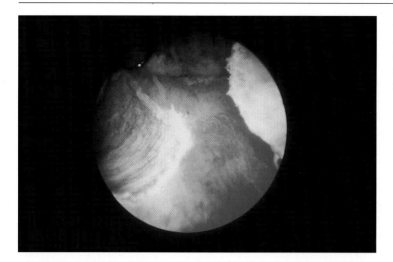

Figure 35.9 *The electrosurgical loop has been passed demonstrating a chip and the circular fibres of the myometrium underneath.*

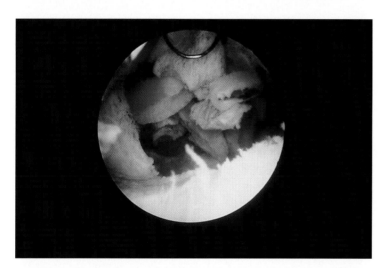

Figure 35.10 *After each chip is cut it is pushed to the fundus.*

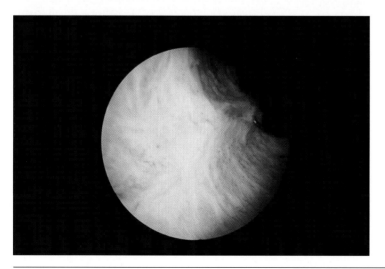

Figure 35.11 *An island of endometrial tissue is left remaining which should be excised.*

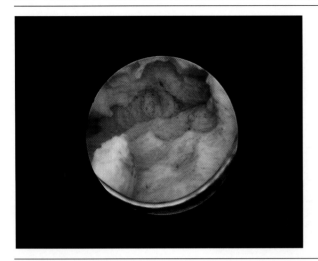

Figure 35.12 *The completed uterine cavity after the resection.*

ROLLERBALL ELECTROABLATION

This is a technique which is commoner in the North America and Australia than in Europe and relies on the modified urological resectoscope fitted with a ball electrode which is moved across the endometrial surface whilst a blended cutting current is used to cause tissue blanching and destruction. It is important to ensure that the endometrial thickness is no more than 3–4 mm at the time of surgery, and this can be achieved by pretreatment with a GnRH analogue or by curettage. Complications are similar to those encountered with TCRE but the chance of uterine perforation is less although not an impossibility. The results of rollerball electroablation are similar to those achieved at TCRE but submucous fibroids cannot be resected and as with laser endometrial ablation there is no specimen for histological analysis. Endometrial sampling before the procedure is mandatory.

LASER ABLATION

Goldrath first described laser endometrial ablation in 1981. The neodymium–yttrium–aluminium–garnet (Nd-YAG) laser is most suitable to laser photocoagulation of the endometrium in view of the fact it is not absorbed by fluids and its tissue penetration, of 4–5 mm is ideally suited to hysteroscopic surgery.

Instrumentation and preoperative preparation

It is essential that the laser equipment is regularly maintained and a dedicated laser technician is in charge and assists the surgeon during the procedure. The Nd-YAG flexible quartz laser fibre is carried in a multichannel hysteroscope with a continuous flow irrigation system. The power output required is usually between 30 and 80 W. As with TCRE, the use of a hysteroscopic infusion pump ensures adequate uterine distension and accurate control over distension pressures. The fluid used for uterine distension can be a physiological solution such as normal saline as there is no concern regarding the use of electrolyte. Consequently, concerns regarding hyponatraemia and cerebral encephalopathy associated with glycine solution are avoided. However, fluid overload with cardiac failure can still occur, and as the surgery tends to be slower than with TCRE, fluid balance can be more difficult to maintain. Pharmacological endometrial preparation is essential before laser endometrial ablation to ensure that the full thickness of the endometrium is destroyed during surgery.

Procedure

As in TCRE, it is best to treat the areas around the tubal ostia and the fundus first. The quartz laser fibre is drawn towards the sheath at the same time as the laser is activated. The commonest laser technique is the "dragging" technique with the laser fibre in contact with the endometrium to develop several furrows down to the myometrium. The "blanching" technique is achieved by holding the fibre a short distance away from the endometrium and "painting" it across the surface. The depth of destruction achieved with this technique is less than in the contact mode and in a pretreated patient the endometrium can look quite pale and hence definition of treated and untreated areas can be difficult. Close monitoring of fluid balance is essential and the operation must be terminated if the fluid absorbed is greater than 1.5–2 litres.

Results

The results of laser endometrial ablation are similar to endometrial resection and roller-ball endometrial ablation. Garry *et al.* reported on 524 women who had undergone Nd-YAG laser ablation with a mean follow-up of 15 months. The data were not subjected to life-table analysis, but 14.3% of women required a repeat procedure and 6.8% of women had a subsequent hysterectomy. At follow-up, 28.9% of women were amenorrhoeic, and of the remainder 93.1% reported a decrease in subjective menstrual volume and 58.9% a reduction in their symptom of dysmenorrhoea.

Complications and their prevention

As with rollerball ablation, one major drawback of laser ablation is the absence of a histological specimen of the treated tissue and consequently thorough endometrial sampling must be performed preoperatively.

Operative complications are similar to those of TCRE although it is felt that uterine perforation is less common. Problems peculiar to patients in the laser group are the potential dangers inherent in laser energy.

OTHER TECHNIQUES OF ENDOMETRIAL ABLATION

In an effort to overcome the need for training and technical skills associated with hysteroscopic methods of endometrial destruction, even less invasive techniques of ablation are under development. Phipps *et al.* have developed a technique of radiofrequency-induced thermal endometrial ablation leading to a reduction in menstrual flow, but unfortunately two grossly obese women developed vesicovaginal fistulae. This problem has since been surmounted by the use of an extra large vaginal guard. Sharp *et al.* has used microwaves to cause endometrial heating down to a depth of 6 mm. No grounding is required with this technique and uterine temperature is continuously monitored and controlled by the surgeon via a foot switch. The probe is "painted" over the endometrium keeping the temperature reading in the range 80–95°C for 2–3 min. A total of 23 women have been treated after endometrial pretreatment of whom 57% were amenorrhoeic at six month follow-up. About 13% of women required retreatment after inadequate endometrial preparation and an overall success rate of 96% was reported with 80% of women reporting complete relief from dysmenorrhoea. There were no reported complications.

Other techniques that have been developed include thermal balloons which are introduced into the uterine cavity, a computer-controlled continuously circulating hot irrigating system, cryoablation and endometrial ablation by photodynamic therapy to destroy the endometrium after exposure to a photosensitizer. All these techniques appear promising as they avoid the operative complications described above and do not rely on operator skill. However, all these techniques suffer from the fact that most are blind procedures and consequently they run the risk of the development of a "false passage" and of unrecognized uterine perforation.

SUGGESTED READING

Chullapram T, Song JY, Fraser IS: Medium-term follow-up of women with menorrhagia treated by rollerball endometrial ablation. *Obstet Gynecol* 1996 **88**: 71–76.

Garry R, Shelley-Jones D, Mooney P, Phillips G: Six hundred laser ablations. *Obstet Gynecol* 1995 **85**: 24–29.

Hart R, Magos AL: Endometrial ablation. *Curr Opin Obstet Gynaecol* 1997 **9**: 226–232.

O'Connor H, Magos AL: Endometrial resection for the treatment of menorrhagia. *N Engl J Med* 1996 **335**: 151–156.

Phipps JH, Lewis, BV, Roberts T, Prior MV, Hand JW, Elder M, Field SB: Treatment of functional menorrhagia by radiofrequency-induced thermal endometrial ablation. *Lancet* 1990 **335**: 374–376.

Sharp NC, Cronin N, Feldberg I, Evans M, Hodgson D, Ellis S: Microwaves for menorrhagia: a new fast technique for endometrial ablation. *Lancet* 1994 **346**: 1003–1004.

36

HYSTEROSCOPIC RESECTION OF UTERINE SEPTUM

Rafael F. Valle

Approximately 20% of women with a uterine anomaly, particularly those with uterine septum have recurrent abortions. The anomaly is due to a lack of reabsorption of an original septum that results from a fusion of two Mullerian ducts in the mid portion. The resulting septum is usually avascular and composed of fibrotic tissue. Consequently, when implantation occurs at this site, the blastocyst may not receive sufficient blood supply resulting in a miscarriage. The decreased uterine volume by this septation may also contribute to repetitive abortions in early pregnancy and malpositions in the third trimester of pregnancy. The diagnosis is obtained with a hysterosalpingogram (Fig. 36.1) and when symptomatic the uterine septum is best treated by hysteroscopy.

Uterine septa may be of different lengths and widths involving only the corporeal portion of the uterus or extending to the cervix. Occasionally there is also septation of the vagina.

PROCEDURE

Hysteroscopic metroplasty

Hysteroscopy is best done immediately after menstruation. This timing is done to avoid debris, mucus or a thickened endometrium that may impair visualization and make the operation more difficult. The procedure is performed under general

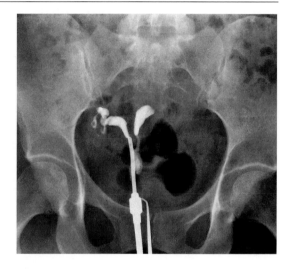

Figure 36.1 *Hysterosalpingogram shows a divided uterine cavity.*

anaesthesia and under endotracheal intubation with a concomitant laparoscopy. First, laparoscopy is performed to outline the external contour of the uterus and to assess tubal integrity. An operative hysteroscope with a 7-mm outer diameter is used. A continuous flow system allowing constant washing of the uterus is preferable particularly when hysteroscopic scissors are utilized. This is the most common method to treat uterine septum, as the tissue is avascular and it permits direct cutting with minimal bleeding. The corporeal septum is outlined after complete hysteroscopic evaluation of both uterine cavities utilizing an electrolyte–low viscosity fluid (Ringer's lactate, normal saline, dextrose 5% in half-normal saline). Using semi-rigid 7 French hysteroscopic scissors, the septum is divided on the midline. This is to avoid blood vessels that may cross and arch close to the uterine wall. The septal division is done systematically from side to side until both uterotubal cones and tubal ostia are seen (Figs 36.2–36.4). A surgical assistant observes the transillumination of the hysteroscopic light through the uterine wall with a dimmed light or no light from the laparoscope. The transillumination becomes one and uniform after complete division of the septum unifying the two uterine cavities. At the completion of the procedure, the intrauterine pressure is decreased to below 60 mmHg. By decompression, arterial bleeding usually at the fundal region can be visualized. Selective coagulation is then performed utilizing a ball-tip electrode after switching to a non-electrolyte distending medium (glycine, sorbitol or mannitol).

Metroplasty with a resectoscope

When a broad septum is encountered, a resectoscope can be used (Figs 36.5 and 36.6). This may expedite the procedure and permits simultaneous cutting and coagulation. Using a special thin angled electrosur-

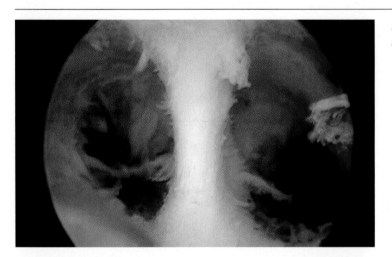

Figure 36.2 Uterine septum as seen by hysteroscopy.

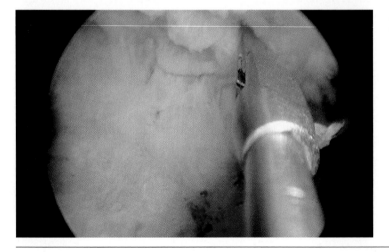

Figure 36.3 Division of septum with hysteroscopic scissors.

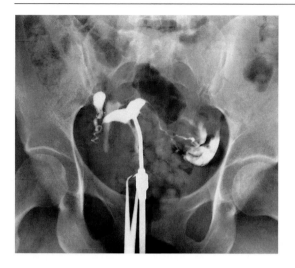

Figure 36.4 Hysterosalpingographic view of uterine cavity after treatment of the septum.

gical knife applied to the tissue with gentle pressure, continuous cutting from side to side is done. The procedure performed is similar to that with scissors. Only fluids devoid of electrolytes can be used (glycine 1.5%, sorbitol 3%, or mannitol 5%). In the presence of electrolytes, erratic dispersion of electricity occurs leading to poor cutting and coagulating effects. An unmodulated current of 90–100 W blended with a modulated current of 30–40 W is most useful. A fiberoptic laser, especially the Nd:YAG laser fitted with a sculpted sharp-tip and activated at 25–30 W can also be used. Because lasers are not conductive, electrolyte–low viscosity fluids can be utilized.

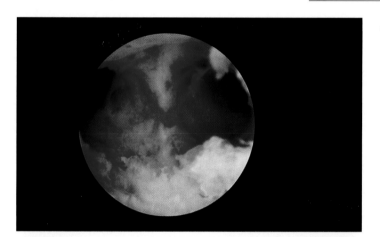

Figure 36.5 Hysteroscopic view of wide uterine septum.

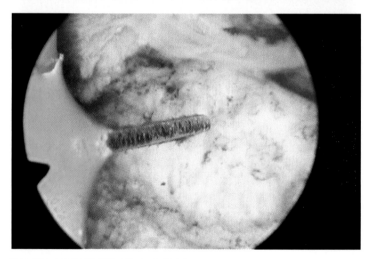

Figure 36.6a

Figure 36.6b

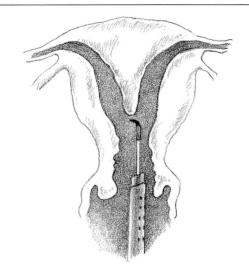

Figure 36.6c

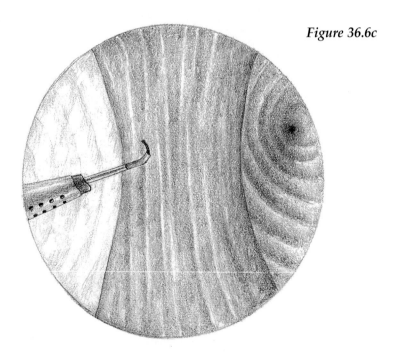

Figures 36.6a, 36.6b, 36.6c *Division of septum with resectoscopic electrical knife.*

It is important to measure precisely the liquids delivered into the uterine cavity and the liquids recovered. This is to avoid the possibility of excessive intravasation of fluids.

Resection of uterine septum extending to the cervix

Uterine septum may extend down to the cervix. Sometimes a concomitant vaginal septum is also found (Fig. 36.7). Here, the

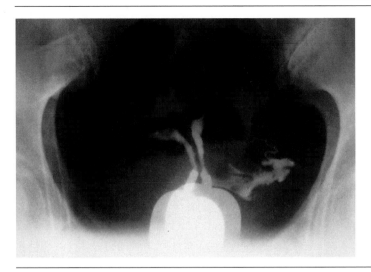

Figure 36.7 *Hysterosalpingogram demonstrates uterine septum with septate cervix.*

vaginal septum is first removed. For the hysteroscopic part, a uterine probe or an indwelling catheter is introduced into one of the divided cervical canals. This is done after the opposite canal has been dilated for insertion of an operative hysteroscope. The probe or indwelling catheter is placed just above the internal cervical os to obtain a slight indentation of the septum at this level. Under hysteroscopic view, a small fenestration is performed with semirigid hysteroscopic scissors (Figs 36.8–36.10) The probe is then inserted through this window and the indwelling catheter is permitted to protrude slightly through the window. After sufficient space has been created to view the opposing uterine cavity, the probe or the catheter is withdrawn. The corresponding endocervical canal is occluded with a tenaculum or the indwelling catheter is inflated slightly to occlude the cervical canal. Hysteroscopic division of the corporeal uterine septum is then started. The septum is progressively divided until symmetry of the uterine cavity is achieved at the fundal area, and the uterotubal cones and the tubal ostia are seen. The uterine cavity is observed systematically from the internal cervical os to assure complete division of the septum. Usually, the uterine septum, at the level just above the internal os, is very thin. Perhaps this is because of the embryological reabsorption that usually begins in this area,

thus facilitating the initial hysteroscopic fenestration of the septum. The resectoscope or the fiber-laser can also be used in the treatment of uterine septum.

POSTOPERATIVE TREATMENT

Postoperatively, the patients are treated with oestrogen such as Premarin, orally 2.5 mg twice daily for 30 days. Medroxyprogesterone acetate (Provera) 10 mg daily orally is added during the last ten days of the Premarin cycle. This hormonal treatment is to artificially stimulate overgrowth of endometrium over the raw area left by the resection. A hysterosalpingogram is repeated at the completion of hormonal therapy to assess the symmetry of the uterine cavity and the complete resection of the septum. If this examination is normal the patient is allowed to conceive.

POTENTIAL COMPLICATIONS AND THEIR PREVENTION

The most significant complications are uterine perforation, fluid overload, and postoperative bleeding.

Uterine perforation

This can occur with any of the three methods used. Nonetheless, following a

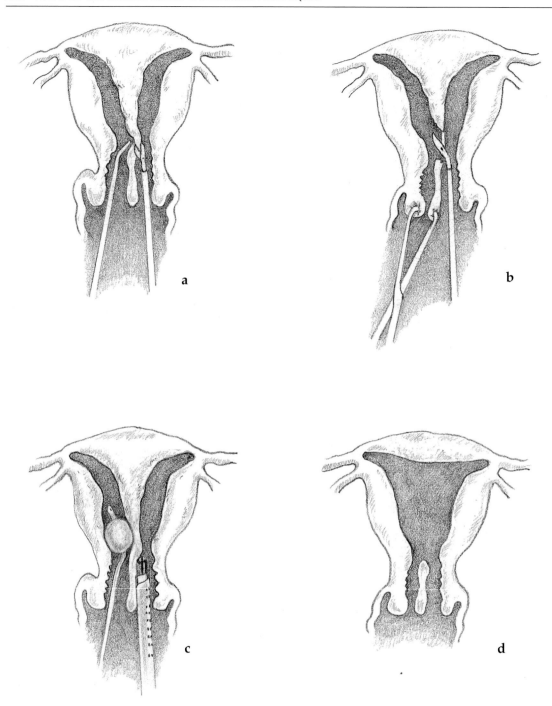

Figure 36.8 *Hysteroscopic metroplasty of complete uterine septum with septate cervix. **a** Fenestration done at level of internal cervical os using scissors. **b** The cervical canal not housing the hysteroscope is occluded and the corporeal septum divided. **c** An indwelling catheter is used to facilitate initial septal fenestration. Here the use of an electrode is demonstrated. **d** Uterine cavity after hysteroscopic metroplasty for complete septum with septate cervix. The cervical portion is not removed.*

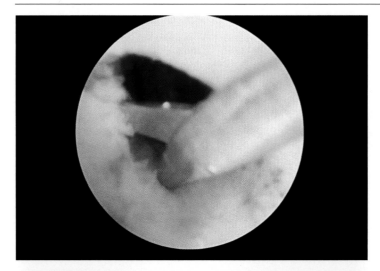

Figure 36.9 Initial hysteroscopic fenestration of septum.

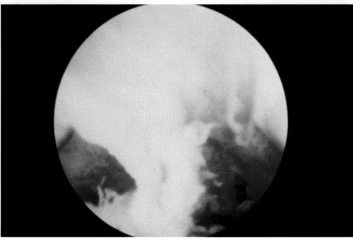

Figure 36.10 Completed septal fenestration.

systematic approach to dissection and monitoring, this complication can be avoided. When using scissors, observe the small arterioles at the juxtaposed myometrium of the uterine fundus. This alerts the hysteroscopist to stop the procedure before entering the myometrium. When using electrosurgery, this landmark may be lost due to the coagulation of the tissue. However, the symmetry of both uterotubal cones, the transillumination seen by the laparoscopist, and the recognition of the anatomic landmarks of the uterus should suffice to prevent this complication. As with electrosurgery, when using a fiber-optic laser, particular attention should be given to the myometrial junction.

Fluid overload

This is crucial especially when using electrolyte-free fluid. It is important to maintain the intrauterine pressure at <100 mmHg. Intake and output of the fluid should be monitored carefully. The surgeon should not allow a deficit of more than 800–1000 ml when using electrolyte-free fluids or more than 1500–2000 ml when using fluids containing electrolytes. Urine output should also be measured. Prophylactic diuretics can be used if large deficits are encountered. The continuous monitoring of pulse oximetry, oesophageal temperature and vital signs by the anaesthesiologist will also assure that early signs of fluid overload can be detected. This is particularly important when the procedure is done under general anaesthesia.

Postoperative bleeding

This can occur particularly when using mechanical scissors. The precaution of decreasing the intrauterine pressure just before completing the operation and observing for any arterial bleeding should be done.

CONTRAINDICATIONS

There are few contraindications to hysteroscopic resection of uterine septum. Most are related to lack of indication or other associated problems that may preclude endoscopic procedure either by laparoscopy or hysteroscopy. These include a bicornuate uterus, a didelphic uterus, recent pelvic inflammatory disease, and relative contraindications such as in a patient with unproven fertility. Also, lack of proper instrumentation is a contraindication.

CONCLUSIONS

Hysteroscopic metroplasty is the treatment of choice for symptomatic septate uterus. After the procedure, the reproductive outcome of women with habitual abortion is markedly improved with a reported viable pregnancy rate of 85–90%. Some infertile women, particularly those who require expensive treatments for ovulation induction, insemination, or *in vitro* fertilization may also benefit from prophylactic removal of a uterine septum. The routine treatment of uterine septum in women who have not proven their fertility, however, does not seem to be warranted.

SUGGESTED READING

Hysteroscopic metroplasty. In Siegler AM, Valle RF, Lindemann HJ, Mencaglia L: *Therapeutic Hysteroscopy. Indications and Techniques.* C.V. Mosby, St Louis, 1990, pp. 62–81.

Fedele L, Arcaini L, Parazzini F *et al.*: Reproductive prognosis after hysteroscopic metroplasty in 102 women: live-table analysis. *Fertil Steril* 1993 **59**: 768.

Hassiakos DK, Sourlas BA: Transcervical division of the uterine septa. *Obstet Gynecol Surv* 1990 **45**: 165.

Siegler AM, Valle RF: Therapeutic hysteroscopic procedures. *Fertil Steril* 1988 **50**: 685.

Valle RF: Uterine septa. In Bieber EJ and Loffer FD (eds) *Gynecologic Resectoscopy.* Blackwell Science. Cambridge, Massachusetts, 1995, pp. 128–152.

Valle RF: Septa and synchiae. In Gordon AG, Lewis BV and DeCherney AH (eds) *Atlas of Gynaecologic Endoscopy* 2nd edn. Mosby-Wolfe, London, Baltimore, Chicago, Philadelphia, St Louis, Sydney, Tokyo, 1995, pp. 209–217.

37

HYSTEROSCOPIC TUBAL CANNULATION

Jennifer Y. Claman and Alan H. DeCherney

About 15% of married couples in the United States experience infertility. Tubal disease is the cause of 25–30% of female infertility. Approximately 20% of tubal disease is secondary to proximal tubal occlusion. Traditionally, therapeutic options for these patients included microsurgical resection of the obstruction with reanastomosis or *in vitro* fertilization. Microsurgical resection involves general anaesthesia and a laparotomy resulting in significant patient discomfort and convalescent period. Resected portions of the fallopian tube occasionally fail to demonstrate any histological abnormality, or are found to contain amorphous proteinaceous material without anatomic abnormality. This procedure results in a 40–50% first-year probability of conception under the best of circumstances. *In vitro* fertilization is time consuming, inconvenient to the patient, and results in only an approximate 20% clinical pregnancy rate per attempt. Additional procedures are required for subsequent pregnancies.

Development of a minimally invasive, more convenient technique to restore tubal patency began with interest in transcervical/transuterine tubal sterilization. This technique never achieved acceptable contraceptive efficacy, but provoked interest in transcervical uterine and tubal exploration. Since the mid 1980s a variety of techniques and instruments have been developed for cannulation of the fallopian tube.

STAGES IN THE PROCEDURE

Several catheter designs have been successfully used to recanalize occluded fallopian tubes. Catheter selection appears to depend on the operator's familiarity, and the availability of equipment. Most systems in use today involve the use of co-axial catheters introduced into the fallopian tube in a manner similar to that developed for blood vessels.

Hysteroscopic tubal cannulation

1. Hysteroscopic tubal cannulation is usually done with concurrent laparoscopy. The cervix is grasped with a tenaculum and the cervical canal dilated to accommodate a size 6 Hegar dilator. An operating hysteroscope is introduced into the uterine cavity. The procedure described by Novy and colleagues used CO_2 as the distending medium.
2. A tubal cannulation set is introduced through the hysteroscope. It consists of a 30-cm long 5.5-Fr clear Teflon catheter with a metal obturator. A Y adapter with Luerlock hubs is attached to its proximal end. One arm of the Y adapter is used for irrigation fluid or dye injection and is sealed when not in use. Through the second arm, a 3-Fr catheter tapered to 2.5-Fr at its distal 3 cm is introduced. A steel guidewire, 0.018 in (0.45 mm) diameter is

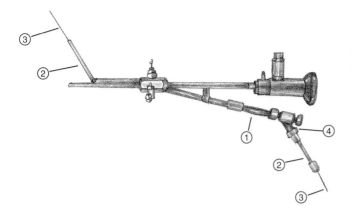

Figure 37.1 Hysteroscopic tubal cannulation system: (1) 5.5-Fr catheter, (2) 3-Fr catheter, (3) steel guidewire, (4) irrigation port of Y adapter.

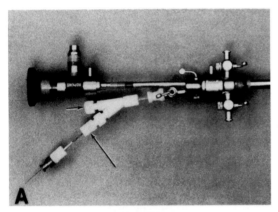

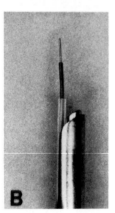

Figure 37.2 **(A)** Hysteroscopic tubal cannulation system. The Teflon cannula is fitted with a Y adapter. The irrigation channel is indicated by a short arrow. The second arm has a Luer lock providing a seal around the 3-Fr inner cannula and guidewire (long arrow). **(B)** Distal end of a rigid hysteroscope with a 3-Fr catheter and guidewire in place. Reproduced from Novy et al. Fertil Steril 1988 **50:** 435.

placed through the lumen of the 3-Fr catheter (Figs 37.1–37.3).

3. The tubal ostium is visualized hysteroscopically, and the 5.5-Fr catheter is guided to the cornual orifice under direct hysteroscopic visualization. The 3-Fr catheter and guidewire are then advanced with the wire protruding slightly. The flexibility of the guide wire is altered by varying the length of the guidewire protruding from the 3-Fr catheter. Lengthening the amount of wire protruding increases the wire flexibility (Fig. 37.4).

4. The guidewire is advanced into the isthmus or until significant resistance is met. The 3-Fr catheter is then advanced over the guidewire until similar resistance is encountered. The guidewire is withdrawn and dye or contrast is injected through the catheter. Tubal patency is evaluated by observing laparoscopic spill of material into the peritoneal cavity, or by performing a postprocedure hysterosalpingogram (Fig. 37.5).

5. If more distal obstruction is encountered, attempts can be made to disimpact it by using the flexible guide wire. By varying the length of the protruding guide wire to attain desired stiffness and moving the wire in a gentle back and forth motion, tubal debris can be dislodged and tubal patency restored.

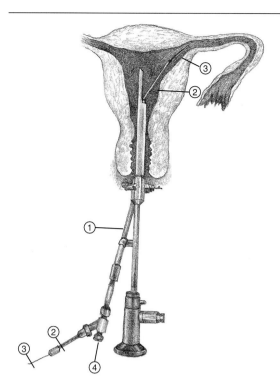

Figure 37.3 *Hysteroscopic tubal cannulation catheter in place: (1) 5.5-Fr catheter, (2) 3-Fr catheter, (3) steel guidewire, (4) irrigation port of Y adapter.*

Balloon tuboplasty

A further modification of the above described system was developed by borrowing from the technology of balloon dilatation of peripheral blood vessels. This procedure is performed under fluoroscopy, intravenous sedation and paracervical block, unless performed in conjunction with laparoscopy, and involves balloon dilatation of obstructed fallopian tubes.

1. The cervix is grasped with a tenaculum. A double balloon catheter is inserted into the lower uterine segment. The first balloon is inflated distal to the cervical os, traction is applied to wedge the catheter against the internal os, and the proximal balloon is inflated sealing the cervical canal.

2. Water-soluble radio-opaque contrast is injected through this catheter to reconfirm proximal tubal occlusion.

3. A 2.5-mm catheter is advanced through the primary catheter and directed into the cornual angle under fluoroscopic guidance.

4. The balloon tuboplasty catheter is then advanced through the catheter wedged in the cornual angle thereby entering the fallopian tube. The balloon tuboplasty catheter consists of a 1-mm shaft through which runs a 0.6-mm guidewire. The tuboplasty catheter is advanced up to the obstruction and the balloon surrounding the shaft is inflated with up to 5 atm with either contrast medium or saline solution. Tubal dilatation is performed until contrast material injected through an accessory port in the balloon tuboplasty catheter confirms tubal patency. When needed, the guidewire is advanced into the strictured area, then the balloon tuboplasty catheter is tracked over the wire allowing balloon dilatation of the obstructed area. An obvious drawback of this technique is exposure of the ovaries to radiation (Figs 37.6–37.9).

POTENTIAL COMPLICATIONS AND THEIR PREVENTION

1. Perforation of the fallopian tube is reported in up to 10% of attempted procedures. The acute angle at the isthmic uterine junction is the area that presents the most difficulty during attempted cannulation. Care must be taken to recognize anatomical variations of patients in this area. The use of flexible catheters to negotiate these curves may decrease the risk of perforation. When perforation occurs, it is left to heal spontaneously, these perforations have no known clinical manifestation.

2. Mild vasovagal reactions have been described during uterine instrumentation and may require atropine treatment. These reactions usually do not preclude

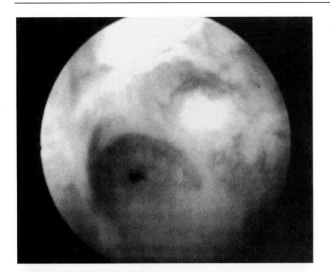

Figure 37.4a

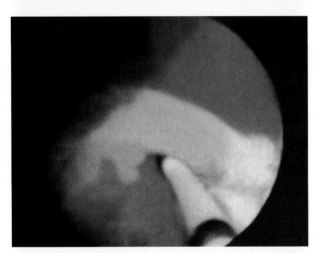

Figure 37.4b

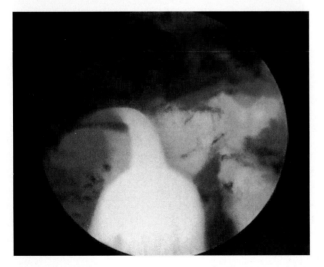

Figure 37.4c

Figures 37.4a to 37.4c *Hysteroscopic view during cannulation. **a** Uterotubal junction. **b** Selective ostial cannulation of the fallopian tube. **c** Tubal cannulation using coaxial catheters.*

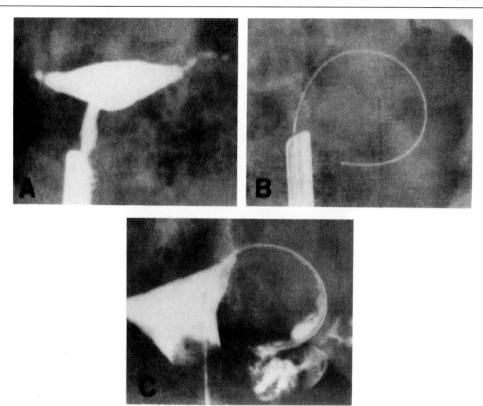

Figures 37.5a to 37.5c *Hysteroscopic cannulation and resolution of obstruction with subsequent peritoneal spillage. **a** Conventional hysterosalpingogram demonstrating proximal tubal occlusion: **b** Hysteroscopic cannulation of the tube with guidewire in the isthmic-ampullary segment. **c** Verification of intratubal guidewire placement and tubal patency by injection of contrast media. Reproduced From Novy et al. Fertil Steril 1988, 438.*

the successful completion of the procedure.

3. Intrauterine/intratubal infection secondary to transvaginal passage of instruments can occur. Strict adherence to aseptic technique is critical to minimize this risk. Pre-procedure cervical culture screening and prophylactic antibiotics are often used.

4. Other potential complications are not specifically related to the cannulation of the fallopian tube, but to the performance of the hysteroscopy. Careful attention to irrigation medium is essential to prevent iatrogenic hyponatraemia when hypotonic solutions are used. Uterine perforation by the hysteroscope has been reported but is unusual.

CONTRAINDICATIONS

1. Transcervical tubal cannulation should not be performed in the presence of known pelvic infection.

2. A markedly distorted uterine cavity may make the procedure technically difficult, and the feasibility of the procedure should be considered carefully under this circumstance.

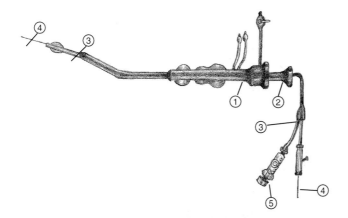

Figure 37.6 *Transcervical balloon tuboplasty catheter. (1) Double balloon catheter, (2) 2.5-mm guiding catheter, (3) balloon angioplasty catheter, (4) steel guidewire, (5) inflation device.*

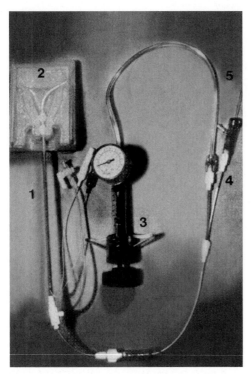

Figure *37.7* *Balloon tuboplasty system: (1) Double balloon introductory catheter, (2) 2.5-mm guiding catheter, (3) manometer syringe, (4) transcervical balloon tuboplasty catheter, (5) steel guidewire preloaded into the main channel of the balloon tuboplasty catheter. Reproduced From Confino et al. JAMA 1990* **264**; *2080.*

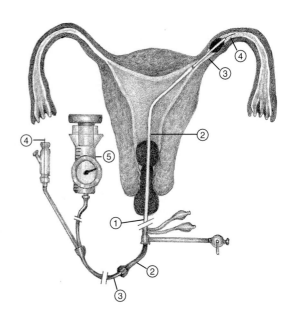

Figure *37.8* *Balloon tuboplasty catheter in place. (1) Double balloon catheter, (2) 2.5-mm guiding catheter, (3) balloon angioplasty catheter, (4) steel guidewire, (5) inflation device. Redrawn From Katz, Chapter 20,* Practical Manual of Operative Laparoscopy and Hysteroscopy, *p. 195.*

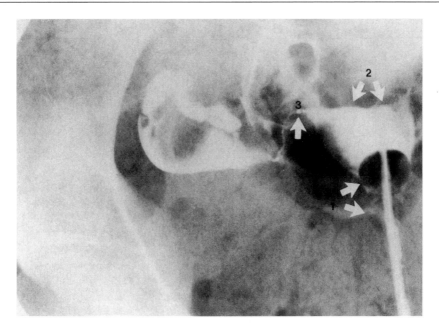

Figure* 37.9** *Hysterosalpingogram demonstrating transcervical balloon tuboplasty system in place following successful balloon dilatation of a cornual obstruction. Peritoneal spill following the injection of radiocontrast material demonstrates tubal patency. (1) Double ballon catheter with two tandem balloons inflated in the lower uterine segment and endocervical canal, (2) guiding catheter wedged in the the cornual angle, (3) balloon marker of the transcervical balloon tuboplasty catheter. Reproduced From Confino, et al. JAMA 1990* **264; 2080.*

3. The procedure should not be attempted in patients with known distal tubal disease. Recannulation of the distal fallopian tube is technically difficult, often unsuccessful, and has not been adequately evaluated. Treatment of proximal tubal disease in the presence of more distal disease may increase the likelihood of developing a distal ectopic pregnancy.

SUGGESTED READING

Confino E, Tur-Kaspa I, DeCherney A *et al.*: Transcervical balloon tuboplasty: a multicenter study. *JAMA* 1990 **264**: 2079–2082.

Flood JT, Grow DR: Transcervical tubal cannulation: a review. *Obstet Gynecol Surv* 1993 **48**: 768–776.

Kumpe DA, Zwerdlinger SC, Rothbarth LJ, Durham JD, Albrecht BH: Proximal fallopian tube occlusion: diagnosis and treatment with transcervical fallopian tube catheterization. *Radiology* 1990 **177**: 183–187.

Novy MJ, Thurmond AS, Patton P, Uchida BT, Rosch J: Diagnosis of cornual obstruction by transcervical fallopian tube cannulation. *Fertil Steril* 1988 **50**: 434–440.

Risquez F, Confino E: Transcervical tubal cannulation, past, present, and future. *Fertil Steril* 1993 **60**: 211–226.

INDEX